ONE Touch

Forensic Medicine & Toxicology

For NEET/NEXT/FMGE/INI-CET

J Magendran MBBS, MD (Forensic Medicine)
Professor
Saveetha Medical College, Saveetha University
Chennai, Tamil Nadu, India

CBSPD
Dedicated to Education

CBS

CBS Publishers & Distributors Pvt Ltd

• New Delhi • Bengaluru • Chennai • Kochi • Kolkata • Lucknow
• Mumbai • Hyderabad • Nagpur • Patna • Pune • Vijayawada

ONE Touch
Forensic Medicine & Toxicology
For NEET/NEXT/FMGE/INI-CET

ISBN: 978-93-94525-55-9

First Edition: 2024

Published by **Satish Kumar Jain** and produced by **Varun Jain** for

CBS Publishers & Distributors Pvt Ltd
4819/XI Prahlad Street, 24 Ansari Road, Daryaganj, New Delhi 110 002, India.
Ph: +91-11-23289259, 23266861, 23266867 Website: www.cbspd.com
Fax: 011-23243014
e-mail: delhi@cbspd.com; cbspubs@airtelmail.in.

Corporate Office: 204 FIE, Industrial Area, Patparganj, Delhi 110 092
Ph: +91-11-4934 4934 Fax: 4934 4935
e-mail: feedback@cbspd.com; bhupesharora@cbspd.com

Branches

- **Bengaluru:** Seema House 2975, 17th Cross, K.R. Road, Banasankari 2nd Stage, Bengaluru-560 070, Karnataka
  Ph: +91-80-26771678/79 Fax: +91-80-26771680 e-mail: bangalore@cbspd.com
- **Chennai:** 7, Subbaraya Street, Shenoy Nagar, Chennai-600 030, Tamil Nadu
  Ph: +91-44-26680620, 26681266 Fax: +91-44-42032115 e-mail: chennai@cbspd.com
- **Kochi:** 68/1534, 35, 36-Power House Road, Opp. KSEB, Cochin-682018, Kochi, Kerala
  Ph: +91-484-4059061-65 Fax: +91-484-4059065 e-mail: kochi@cbspd.com
- **Kolkata:** Hind Ceramics Compound, 1st Floor, 147, Nilganj Road, Belghoria, Kolkata-700056, West Bengal
  Ph: +033-2563-3055/56 e-mail: kolkata@cbspd.com
- **Lucknow:** Basement, Khushnuma Complex, 7-Meerabai Marg (Behind Jawahar Bhawan), Lucknow-226001, Uttar Pradesh
  Ph: +0522-4000032 e-mail: tiwari.lucknow@cbspd.com
- **Mumbai:** PWD Shed, Gala No. 25/26, Ramchandra Bhatt Marg, Next to J.J. Hospital Gate No. 2, Opp. Union Bank of India, Noor Baug, Mumbai-400009, Maharashtra
  Ph: +91-22-66661880/89 Fax: +91-22-24902342 e-mail: mumbai@cbspd.com

Representatives

- **Hyderabad** +91-9885175004
- **Pune** +91-9623451994
- **Patna** +91-9334159340
- **Vijayawada** +91-9000660880

Printed at: Goyal Offset Works Pvt. Ltd.

Preface

'ज्ञानं परमं बलम्' (Gyaanam Paramam Balam)

'Knowledge is the Supreme Power'

Dear Students,

This motto has been the driving force behind my thirst for knowledge. I have been immensely blessed to be in the teaching industry which provides me an opportunity to stay in touch with students on regular basis, and this close association always inspires me to learn more and more each day.

I want to begin by expressing my deep gratitude to all the students. Your questions and suggestions have been invaluable in shaping my teaching approach and my own growth as an educator.

The motivation behind this revision book arises from your consistent requests for a concise resource to swiftly review or fully grasp the concepts of Forensic Medicine. I have spent many months contemplating this idea, and I am thrilled to present you with a condensed version of Forensic Medicine and Toxicology theory that I believe will greatly aid you in your pursuit of excellence. It's not a shortcut but the best tool for fast revision.

What can you expect from this book?

- **Concise Theory (Just 120 pages):** I have condensed the entire content merely in 120 pages by employing a flowchart approach and optimizing page space usage.
- **Important Images:** I have included essential clinical images throughout the book for ease of understanding the concept.
- **Mnemonics:** Text is supplemented with many mnemonics for easy recall.
- **Previous Years Questions:** To aid in quick exam revision, I have included the Previous Years Questions (PYQs) from the last 3 years (NEET PG/FMGE/INI-CET) at the end of the book (up to July 2023).

The students who have already covered Forensic Medicine from any other sources, this concise resource can serve as a rapid revision tool before their exams. This book will prove to be immensely helpful for such students. Memorizing this content alone will suffice for Forensic Medicine. Throughout the book, the content is presented in the form of Flowcharts, Figures, Tables and various boxes for Last-minute revision.

I have put forth my utmost efforts to make this book concise, productive, and error-free. However, if you happen to spot any mistakes, please bring them to my attention by emailing me at drmagi83@yahoo.co.in.

If you wish to connect with me directly, you can find me on Instagram using my handle- drmagendranjfmt

I extend my best wishes to all of you. Sending you lots of love and blessings!

J Magendran

Contents

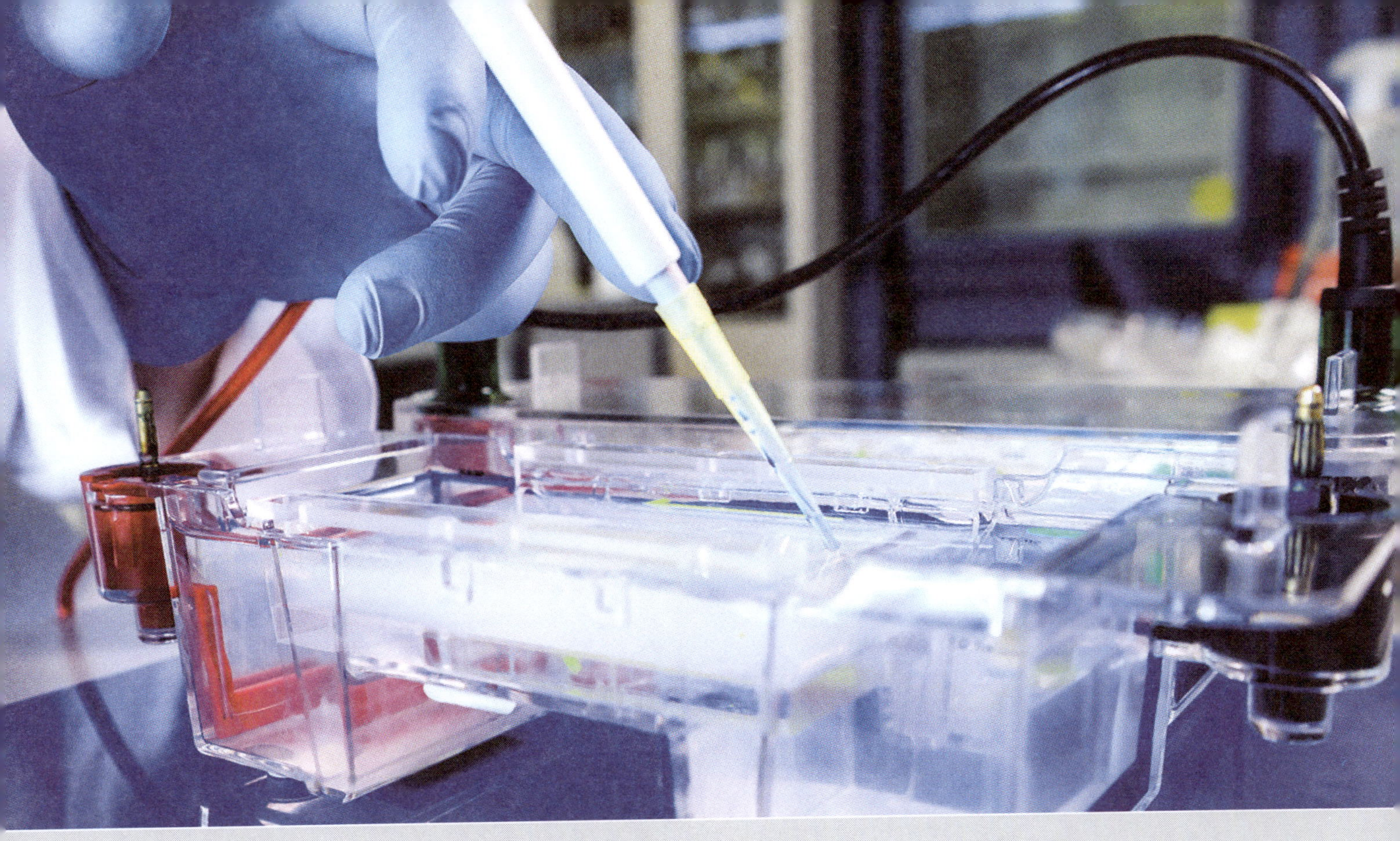

THEORY

1. FORENSIC THANATOLOGY

THANATOLOGY

The **study of death**Q in all its aspects.

TAPHONOMY

The study of the decomposition processes of human remains.

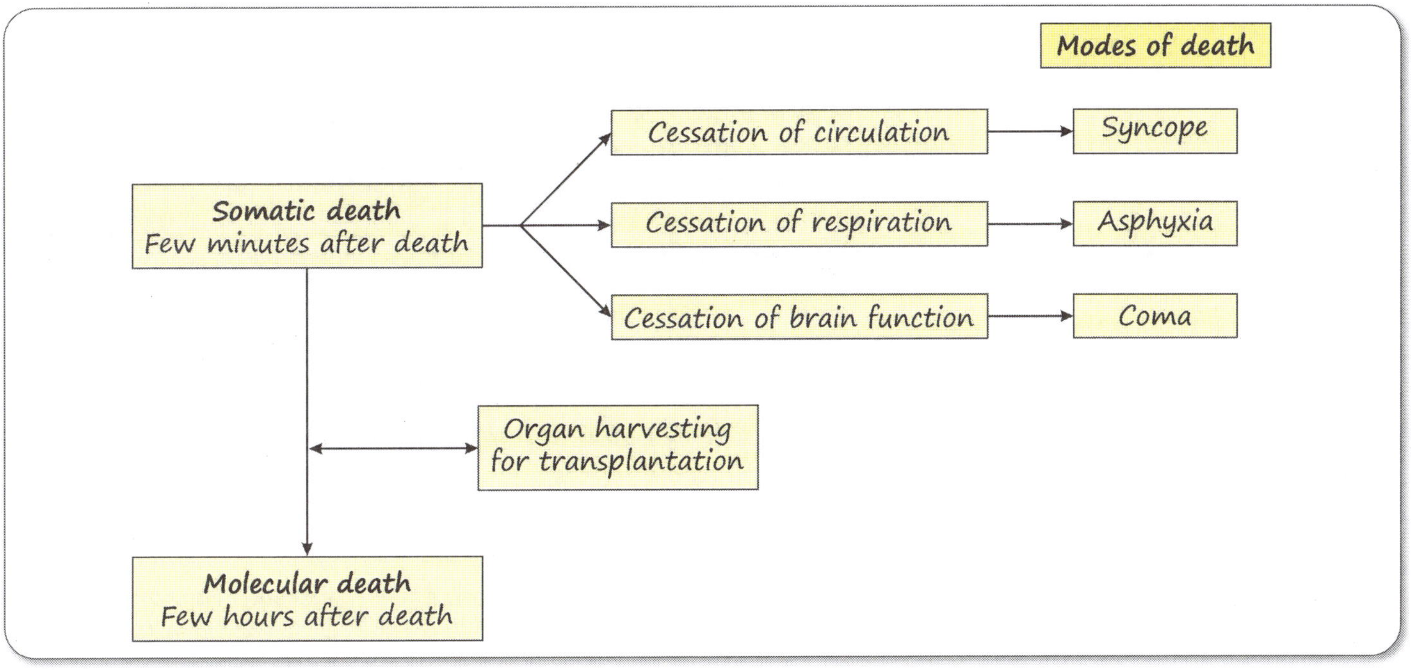

APPARENT DEATH/SUSPENDED ANIMATION

(The person appears to be dead but he/she is not actually dead)
The signs of life are reduced to very minimum that it cannot be detected by routine clinical methods.

Conditions Causing Suspended Animation

Mnemonic:

Suspended Animation IN NEW HD TV

- **In** – Insanity/iatrogenic as in cardiopulmonary surgeries and anesthesia
- **N** – NewbornQ (most common)
- **E** – ElectrocutionQ
- **W** – Wasting diseases like cholera
- **H** – Heat stroke/HypothermiaQ/Hanging
- **D** – DrowningQ/Drugs like barbiturates
- **T** – Typhoid
- **V** – Voluntary (Yoga practitionersQ) (only voluntary cause)

Medicolegal Importance

If death is declared and certified prematurely, in this case the doctor can be punished *for premature declaration of death.*

POSTMORTEM CHANGES

Immediate signs (signs of somatic death)
- Cessation of brain function (insensibility and loss of voluntary power)
- Cessation of respiration
- Cessation of circulation

Early signs (signs of cellular death)
- Pallor and loss of elasticity of skin[Q]
- Primary relaxation of muscles
- Eye changes
- Cooling of body—Algor mortis
- Staining of body—Livor mortis
- Stiffening of body—Rigor mortis

Late signs (signs of cellular death)

Putrefaction
- Autolysis
- Decomposition

Modified form of putrefaction
- Adipocere—moist warm climate
- Mummification—hot dry climate

CHANGES IN THE EYES

- Corneal opacity (in 1 hour)
- Flaccidity of eyeball (**Within half/2 hours after death, I.O.P decreases from 20 mm Hg to 0 mm Hg**)
- **Pupils** (initially dilated, later constricted due to rigor mortis)

Retinal vessels:

Kevorkian sign[Q]**/cattle trucking/railway rucking sign**[Q]

Appearance: Fragmentation or **segmentation of blood columns**[Q] in retinal vessels

Seen by **ophthalmoscope**[Q]

TSD: Appears **within seconds to minutes**[Q] after death, persists till 1 hour. Earliest sign after death in eye[Q]

Sclera: Tache noire sclerotica

If eye lids open

↓

Drying/desiccation, deposition of dust[Q]

↓ 3–6 hours after death

2 triangular opacities on both sides of iris (base on the limbus, apex at the outer canthus) first yellow[Q], then brown and finally black

Vitreous humor: Best medium for time since death[Q]

For TSD, potassium level from vitreous is the best indicator[Q]. (up to 4–5 days after death)

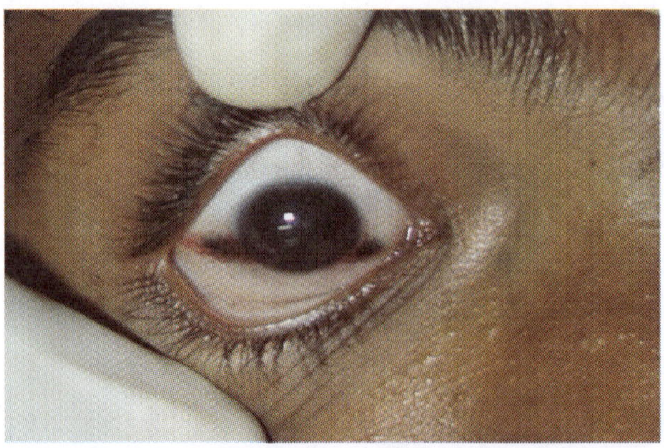

ALGOR MORTIS (CHILL OF DEATH)—POSTMORTEM COOLING OF BODY

- After death, there is a **fall in body core temperature of body**.
- The fall in temperature starts in 15 minutes to ½ hour after death

Sites of measuring core body temperature	**Common sites: Rectum** (8–10 cm above anus)–Except in the case of sodomy **Ideal site: Subhepatic** space **Other sites:** • External auditory meatus (tympanic membrane) • Nose (cribriform plate) • Lower end of the esophagus
Instrument	Chemical thermometer (**thanatometer**)[Q] or electronic thermocouple.

Pattern of Algor Mortis:

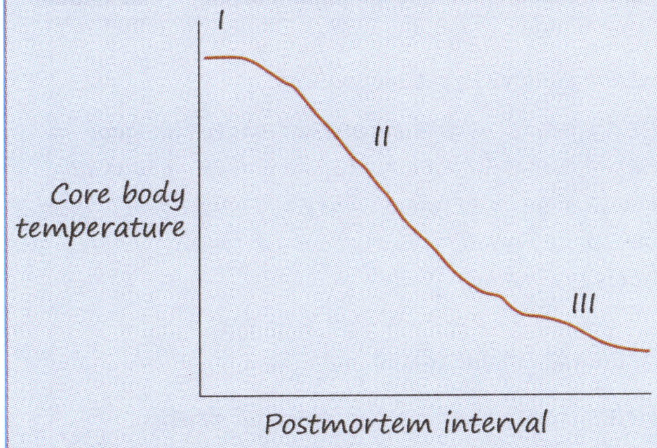

- The curve is sigmoid/inverted
- Three phases:
  1. Phase I: No decrease (isothermic phase)
  2. Phase II: Steep decline in BCT (intermediate phase) (0.4°C–0.7°C/hr)
  3. Phase III: Very gradual decline (terminal phase)

TSD (in hours) =

$$\frac{\textbf{Normal body temperature – Rectal temperature}}{\textbf{Rate of fall of temperature}}$$

Postmortem Caloricity

(Special entity, in which body remains warm for first 2 hours)

- Normally, the body temperature declines after death
- But in this state, the body temperature **does not fall in the initial few hours** after death.

Mechanism (Increased Endogenous Heat Production During Death)

- Disturbed regulation of heat production before death—**Heat stroke**[Q], **Pontine hemorrhage**[Q].
- Heat production due to muscle convulsions—**tetanus, strychnine poisoning**[Q].
- Heat production due to excessive bacterial activity, as in **septicemic**[Q] conditions, cholera and other **fevers**[Q].

LIVOR MORTIS—POSTMORTEM STAINING

Synonyms
- *Lividity*
- *Hypostasis*
- *Cadaveric lividity*
- *Suggillation*[Q]
- *Cogitation*

Mechanism

Cessation of circulation
↓
Stagnation of blood in vessels
↓ ← Gravity
Pooling of blood in capillaries and venules of the dependent parts
↓
Bluish purple staining

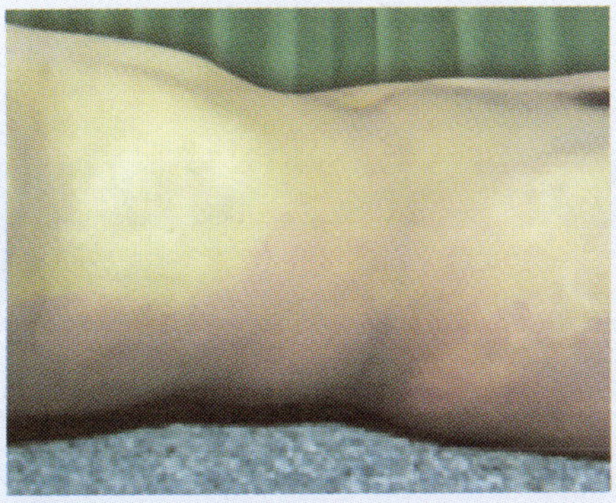

Contd...

Development
Starts as patches in 30 minutes to 2 hour → Patches coalesce with each other to form uniform staining in 4 hours → Complete in 6–12 hours
Fixation of Livor Mortis: 6–12 hours[Q]
Apply pressure → Blanching (not fixed).
Apply pressure → No Blanching (fixed).

Distribution of PM Staining—Depends on the Position of the Body (Dependent Parts)

Supine	Appears in the neck, and the entire back (Exception: Areas directly pressed on the ground)
Prone	It is seen in front
Suspended vertically (as in hanging)	Legs, external genitalia, lower parts of forearms and hands (**Glove and stocking**)[Q]
Submersion in water (drowning)	Face, upper part of the chest, hands, lower arms and feet, as they are the dependent parts
• Running water (drowning in the river) (as the position of the body constantly changes) • Severe anemia • Severe hemorrhage	**No lividity**[Q]

Color of Livor Mortis

Conditions	Color of lividity
Normal	Blue/purplish
Carbon monoxide burns	Cherry red[Q]
Cyanide	Bright red[Q]/Brick red[Q]

Contd...

Conditions	Color of lividity
Hypothermia/refrigeration	Bright pink[Q]
NaCl/nitrite/nitrate/aniline/potassium chlorate/phosphorus/bromates	Chocolate brown[Q]
Aniline	Deep blue
Septic abortion	Bronze
Hydrogen sulphide	Bluish green[Q]

Areas of Pallor in Lividity

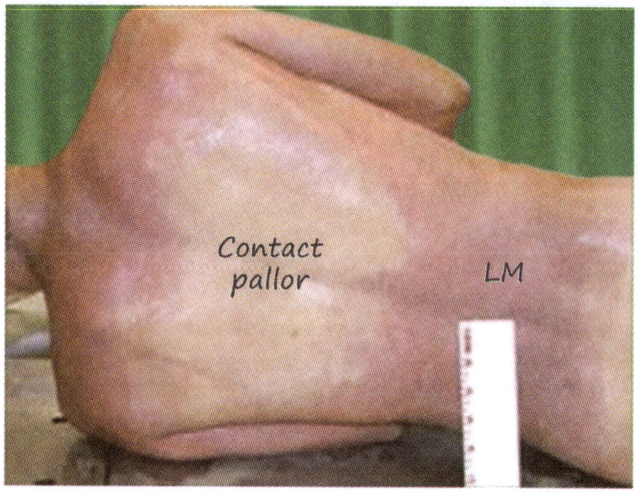

"Contact pallor/Pressure pallor"

- Body parts in **tight contact with the ground** do not show staining.
- Example: Occipital area, shoulder blades, buttocks, posterior aspects of thighs, calves and heels.

Medicolegal Importance

- Helps in estimating the **time of death.**
- Indicates the **posture of the body** at the time of fixation and death.
- Color of lividity may indicate **the cause of death**—poisoning.

RIGOR MORTIS—POSTMORTEM STIFFENING OF MUSCLES

Synonyms

- Cadaveric rigidity
- Postmortem rigor
- Postmortem rigidity
- Postmortem stiffening

- Rigor mortis is state of the muscles becoming stiff or rigid in a dead body.
- **Mechanism:** Due to depletion of ATP stores after death.
- Rigor mortis **begins in 1–2 hours** after the period of primary relaxation.

Rigor mortis is generalized → seen in both voluntary and involuntary muscles.

- **Rigor mortis** begins in 1–2 hours, progresses in 3–4 hours and complete in 6–12 hours.

First seen in: Involuntary muscles	First site of rigor mortis: Myocardium (1 hour)	First external site of rigor mortis: Eyelid

Order of Appearance of Rigor Mortis: Nysten's Rule (1811)

Sequence of Rigor Appearance

- **Myocardium**, eyelids, neck and lower jaw, then face, chest muscles, upper limb, abdomen, lower limb and lastly fingers and toes.
- Rigor mortis disappears in **the same order**[Q] of **appearance** in which it develops.

Rule of 12

- It takes roughly 12 hours to appear.
- Persists for another 12 hours.
- Disappears in another 12 hours.

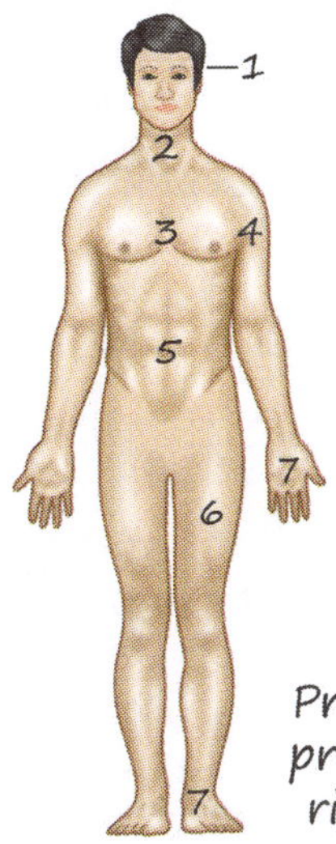

Proximodistal progression of rigor mortis

CONDITIONS SIMULATING (LOOKING LIKE) RIGOR MORTIS

Heat stiffening (burns)	• Heat exposure to body >65°C, stiffness is produced. • **Mechanism:** Muscle protein coagulation[Q] due to heat. **Attitude** • The legs are flexed at the hips and knees, the arms are flexed at the elbows and held out in front of the body and the fingers are hooked like claws.	• Boxer's attitude • Pugilistic attitude • Defense attitude • Fencing attitude
Cold stiffening	• Exposure to freezing temperatures, the tissues become frozen and stiff, simulating rigor. • **Mechanism:** Hardening of the subcutaneous fatty tissue[Q].	
Gas rigidity	Accumulation of decomposing gas in putrefying body.	
Cadaveric spasm (instantaneous rigor) • Firearms in victim's hands in suicides. • Weeds in the hands of victims in drowning.	The **group of voluntary muscles**[Q] goes into a sudden state of stiffening, instead of passing to primary flaccidity after death. **Salient features of cadaveric spasm:** • Seen immediately[Q] after death. • No primary relaxation phase[Q] • Involves only a group of voluntary muscles[Q] (which were in contraction before death). • Exclusively Antemortem[Q] in nature and it cannot be produced artificially[Q]. • Great force[Q] is required to overcome the stiffness.	• **The attitude/last act of the person at the time of death is preserved**[Q]. • **Mechanism:** Unknown[Q], neurogenic

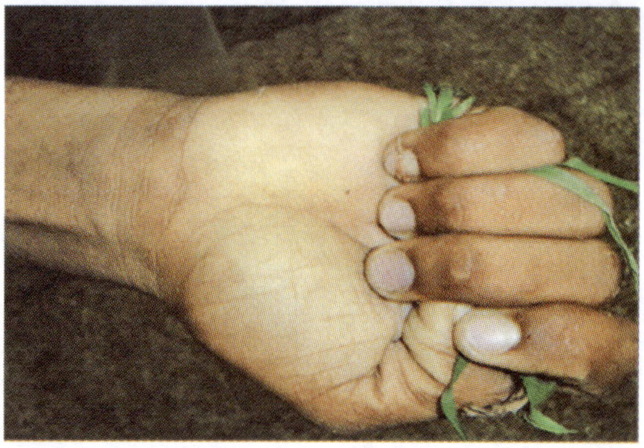

DECOMPOSITION—LATE CHANGES

Autolysis: (auto: self; lysis: breakdown) without bacterial involvement (by lysosomal enzymes)	**Putrefaction** with bacterial involvement. Among these bacteria, clostridium is the chief destructive agent[Q] as it produces **'LECITHINASE[Q]'** enzyme.

Stage of Putrefaction

Putrefaction involves three stages:

1. Color changes
2. Production of gases
3. Colliquative liquefaction of tissues (5–10 days after death[Q])

1. Color Change

- **1st overall site:** Aortic intima—reddish/brownish discoloration.
- **1st external site:** Right iliac fossa—greenish discoloration.
- **Time since death:** Summer—12–18 hours and winter—1–2 days.

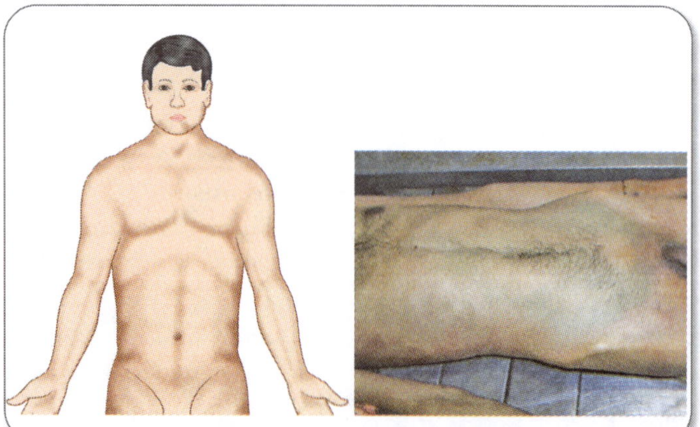

Marbling (Marbled Patterns on the Skin[Q])

- **Areas noted:** Shoulder, roots of the limbs, thighs, sides of abdomen, chest and neck
- **Time:** 36–72 hours[Q].

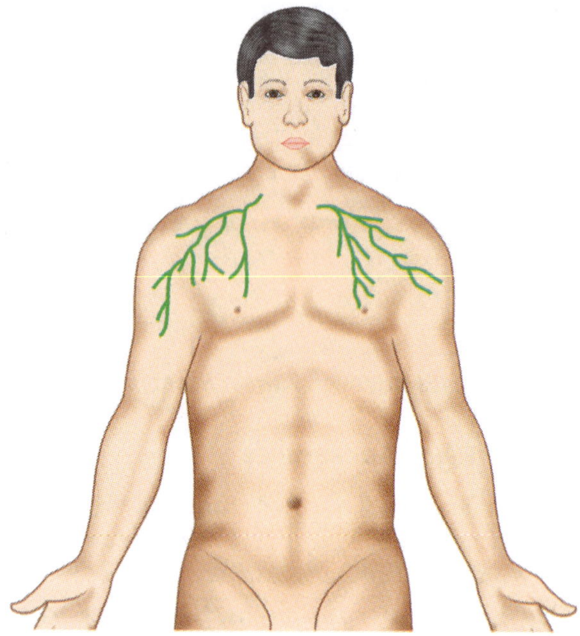

Mechanism

- In putrefaction, when bacteria spread through the blood vessels, hydrogen sulfide gas is formed.
- It results in the conversion of hemoglobin to **sulphmethemoglobin[Q]**
- It caused **greenish staining of inner walls of the vessels[Q]**, a **'marbled' ('road map')**[Q] appearance of the skin.

2. Effects of Gas Formation

- **Gases formed:** Ammonia, carbon dioxide, hydrogen sulfide, phosphorated hydrogen and methane.
- **Principal gas:** Hydrogen sulfide[Q]

Effects	Timeline
Postmortem Skin Blisters Content: gas Base: pale	18–24 hours[Q]
Abdomen gets distended due to the accumulation of gases in the intestines **(gas stiffening[Q])**	18–36 hours

3. Colliquative Putrefaction (Liquefaction)—5–10 Days[Q]

Order of Putrefaction

Earliest	Early	Late	Last
Larynx and trachea	**Mnemonic:** SISter LILLy's Brittle Heart • **SISter:** Stomach, Intestine, Spleen • **Lilly:** Liver • **Brittle:** Brain • **Heart**	• Prostrate • Uterus (nulliparous) • Skin • Tendon	Bone and tooth

Casper's Dictum: Rate of putrefaction in different media

1 week of putrefaction in air = 2 week in water = 8 week in soil.

Air:Water:Earth = 1:2:8

In other words, at a given temperature one week of putrefaction in air is equivalent to two weeks in water and eight weeks buried in soil.

(Fastest in air and slowest on earth)

MODIFIED PUTREFACTION

Adipocere (Grave Wax) **(Hydrolysis and Hydrogenation of Fats)** Commonly seen in **bodies immersed in water**[Q] or in damp warm environment. In this, the fatty tissues of the body change into a substance known as adipocere.	**Mummification** **(Drying and dehydration of the Body)**
• **Sweetish smell**[Q] • Rancid butter smell	Odorless[Q]
Body fat → (Hydrogenation and hydrolysis) → Fatty acids → (Calcium and ammonium ion) → Insoluble soap Warm climate Water (moisture) Clostridium welchi – producing lecithinase Intrinsic lipases **Note:** The process starts by intrinsic lipases, and is continued by bacterial enzymes like lecithinase, which facilitate hydrolysis and hydrogenation	Dead body → Mummification **Dry and hot climate**[Q] Absence of moisture Free circulation of air
• Shortest duration noted in 3 days as well. • Up to 3 months	3 months to 1 year[Q]
Sweetish smell[Q]	Odorless[Q]
• Cause of death[Q]—injuries are preserved • Time since death[Q] • **When involves face, the features are well preserved, helps to** establish the identity	• **Cause of death—injuries are preserved**[Q] • **Time since death**[Q] • **Helps to establish the identity**

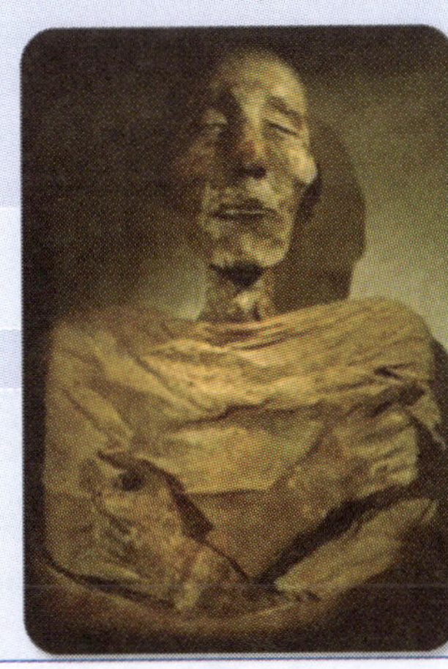

EMBALMING: THANATOPRAXIA

Artificial method of preserving the dead body with antiseptics and preservatives.

Types of embalming:	Embalming fluid		Disadvantages
Arterial: Fluid injected in arteries **Cavity:** Fluid injected in cavities **Surface:** Injection into skin	• **Preservative:** Formalin/Methanol. • **Germicide:** Phenol. and many chemicals **Note:** Ethanol is not a part of embalming solution	**Best time to perform embalming:** Within 6 hours. **Best injection type:** Discontinuous injection and drainage. **Best vessel to inject into:** Carotid/femoral vessels. **Best technique:** High pressure with low flow.	Difficult to interpret injury/diseases[Q]. Alteration of appearance of the body[Q] Dislodgement of thrombi/emboli.

Note:
- **If embalming is done prior to autopsy in poisoning cases,** that amounts to destruction of the evidences (poisons) and **liable to be punished under section** 201 IPC[Q].
- Color of embalmed bodies in Jaundice cases is green.

AUTOPSY (NECROPSY, POSTMORTEM EXAMINATION)

Types

	Medicolegal autopsy most common in India	Clinical/pathological autopsy
Type of deaths	Unnatural deaths	Natural deaths
Authorization	Investigation officer (relatives consent not needed)	Relatives consent mandatory
After autopsy, body handed over to	Investigation officer	Relatives

Virtual autopsy/virtopsy	Psychological autopsy
• Complete imaging of the body through CT/MRI/3D. • To assess the status/disease/injury in the body.	• Done in cases where there is doubt regarding the • Manner of death. • To assess the deceased state of mind before death. • By interviewing relatives and family members.

Obscure autopsy	Negative autopsy
Gross findings are minimal/inconclusive	Gross findings are negative. Negative opinion (No definite opinion can be given even after complete examination and other tests). 2–5% of all autopsies are negative.

First cavity to start: Depends on the dissector choice **(most commonly thorax)**

- **Head injuries:** Cranial cavity.
- **Poisoning cases:** Cranial cavity (to perceive the smell).
- **Newborns:** Abdomen (to determine the level of diaphragm).
- **Asphyxial death**
  - Cranial → Thorax → Abdominal → Neck (last)

- To ensure bloodless dissection, neck should be dissected at last.
- **Pneumothorax:** Thorax
- **Air embolism:** Thorax

Types of Skin Incisions

- **I-shaped incision: (most commonly used)**
  - Incision extending from the chin straight down to the symphysis pubis.
- **Y-shaped incision:**
  - Two incisions each starting from acromion processes, meet in the midline near the xiphisternum and then extend downward straight to pubis.
- **Modified Y-shaped incision:**
  - An incision is made in the midline from the suprasternal notch to the symphysis pubis.
  - It then extends from the suprasternal notch to the mastoid processes on each side.
  - It is used when a detailed study of neck organs is required, like in hanging or strangulation[Q].
- **X-shaped incision:**
  - This incision is made over the back.
  - To demonstrate the deep bruises in custodial death cases.

Techniques of Organ Removal

Organ by organ Virchow's technique	En masse Letulle's technique	Block Ghon's technique	In situ Rokitansky's technique
• Individual organs were **removed one by one**[Q] • Anatomical relations not preserved	• Cervical, thoracic, abdominal and pelvic organs are removed as **en-masse**[Q] (altogether) and organ dissection • **Anatomical relationships preserved and can be studied** • **Rapid technique**	• **Organ blocks**[Q] and organ dissection • Cervical, thoracic, abdominal and urogenital system are removed as organ block (separate blocks)	• **In situ dissection**[Q] of organs • **Fetal brain dissection**[Q] • Infectious diseases like HIV, Hepatitis B

Important Individual Organ Dissection

For solid organs, many parallel cuts, in a fashion similar to slicing a loaf of bread ('**bread loafing**') are done.

Heart dissection: Inflow outflow method[Q]

Following the direction of blood flow.

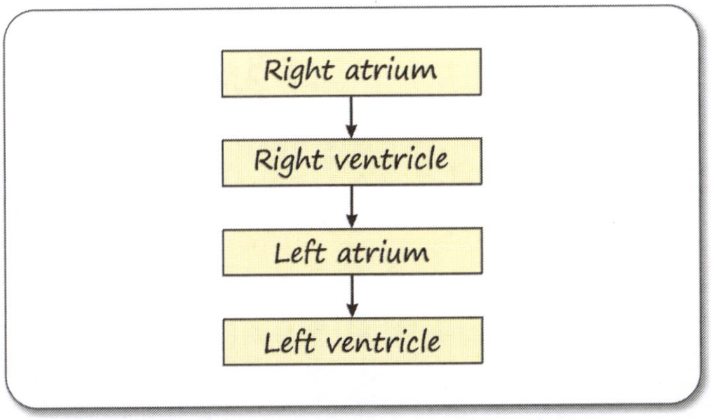

Brain

- In most autopsies, **the brain is examined in the fresh state**[Q].
- In selective cases, the brain is 'fixed' and then examined.
- The **best routine fixative is 10% formalin**[Q] and requires 2–3 weeks for satisfactory fixation.

Spinal Cord

- **Routinely spinal cord is not opened**[Q].
- In cases of suspected spinal injury, spinal cord is opened by **posterior approach**[Q] or anterior approach.

Stomach Dissection (Double Ligation Method)[Q]

- The stomach is removed by cutting between the double ligatures at both ends.
- Then the stomach wall is opened along the greater curvature.

Viscera preservation

Routine viscera preserved during autopsy
- Stomach and its contents
- Upper part of small intestine—30 cm
- Liver (right lobe is preferred)—500 g
- Kidney (half of each kidney)
- Blood 10 mL and urine 100 mL

Preservative not required in
- Hair
- Bone[Q]
- Hair[Q]
- If the viscera analysed in 24 hours
- Refrigeration <4°C

Preservatives

Saturated solution of common salt	Rectified spirit
• Cheap and most commonly[Q] used **Avoided in** • Aconite • Corrosives except carbolic acid	• Best preservative **Avoided in** • Alcohol[Q] • Kerosene[Q] • Phosphorus • Formaldehyde and formic acid[Q]

- **Blood: Sodium fluoride and potassium oxalate**
- **Urine: Thymol, sodium fluoride**
- **Vitreous: Sodium fluoride**
- Virology: 50% glycerol

Note: Formalin is not used[Q] as preservative for chemical analysis because extraction of poison becomes difficult.

Special Organs has to be Sent for Specific Conditions

Viscera preserved	Poisonings
Heart	Strychnine, digitalis[Q]
Brain	Organophosphorus, opiates, carbon monoxide, cyanide, barbiturates.
Spinal cord	Gelsemium, strychnine[Q]
Vitreous	Alcohol (particularly in decomposed bodies[Q])
Lungs	Gaseous poisons
Fatty tissues	Pesticides[Q]
Bone/hair and nail	Heavy metals

2. HUMAN IDENTIFICATION

Determination of the individuality of a person based on physical characteristics.

Parameters for identification of person

Incomplete identification/ presumptive identification	Definitive identification parameter
Race	Tattoo
Sex	Scar
Age	Finger printing—most reliable method
Stature/height	DNA printing—same in monozygotic twins.

Corpus delicti: It is the body of offence or the essence of crime.

- Corpus delicti means facts of any criminal offence.
- The main fact of corpus delicti is the establishment of identity of the dead body, infliction of violence in a particular way, at a particular time and place, by the accused. The case cannot be established unless these are proved.
- If the identity of the victim is not known, it becomes difficult for the police to solve the crime, and therefore the identification of a dead body is essential.

RACE DETERMINATION

- **Bones:** Skull (best), long bones

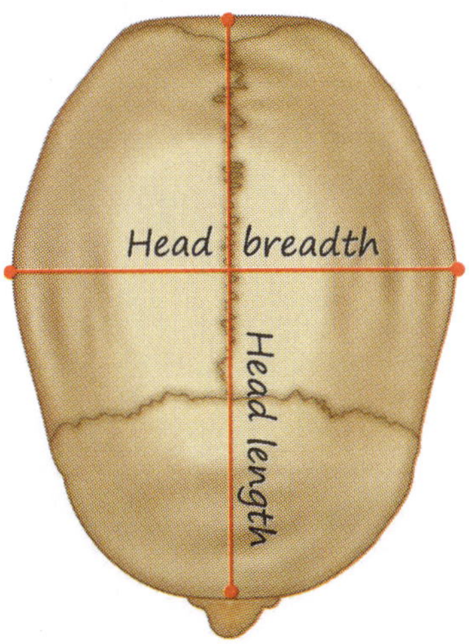

Skull

Mnemonic:

RACE RA (Race) CE (cephalic index)

Cephalic Index[Q] **or cranial index:**

$$\frac{\text{Maximum breath of skull}}{\text{Maximum length of skull}} \times 100$$

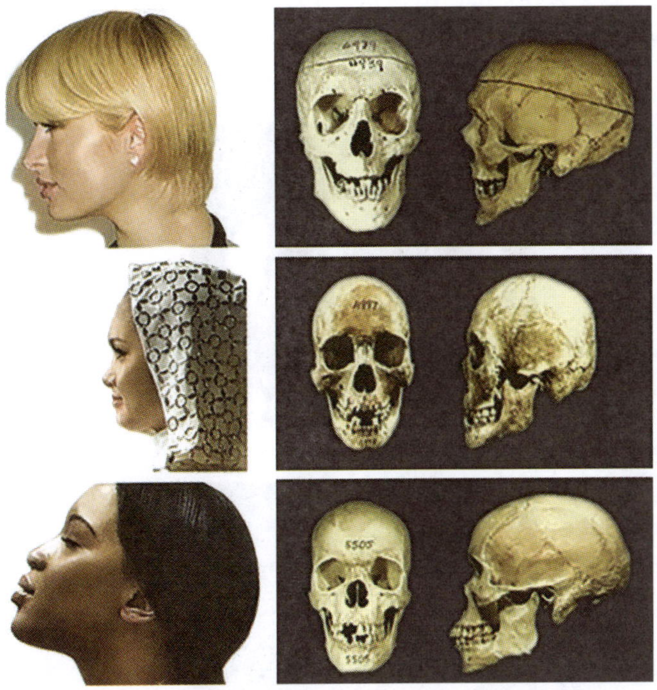

Types	Values	Population
Dolicocephalic	70–74.9	Aryans, Negroes
Mesaticephalic	75–79.9	Europeans, Chinese
Brachycephalic	80–85	Mongolian

- The Indian skull is **Caucasian**[Q] with few Negroid characters.
- Cephalic index of Indian skull: **75–79.9**[Q]**—mesaticephalic**[Q].

Race Determination from Teeth

Mongoloid	Caucasoid	Negroid
• **Shovel-shaped upper central incisors** (posterior surface of the incisors has a central depression centrally with marginal ridges). • **Enamel pearls** (small nodules of enamel). • **Taurodontism** (bull tooth). • The pulp cavity of molars is wide and deep. • The roots are fuse and bent. • **Congenital lack of upper 3rd molars.**	Carabelli's cusp (additional nodule on lingual surface of maxillary molar).	Large teeth with more cusps in their molars with two lingual cusps on mandibular first premolars are common.

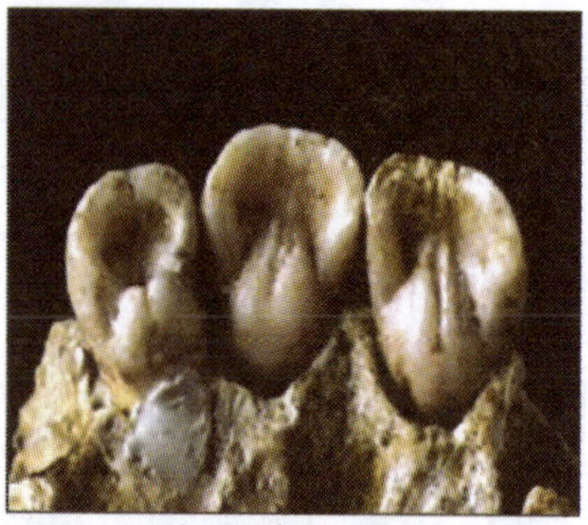
Shovel incisor

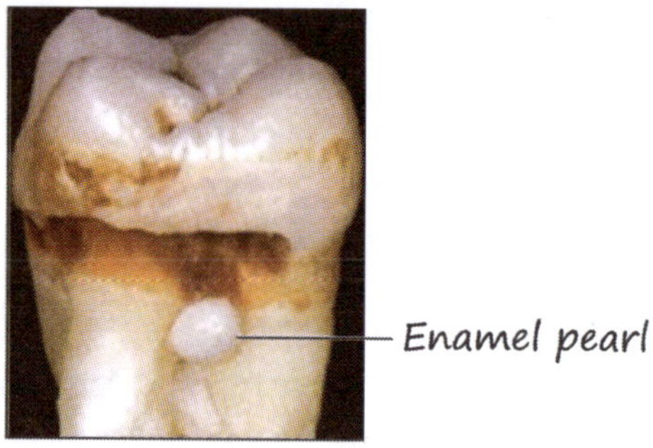

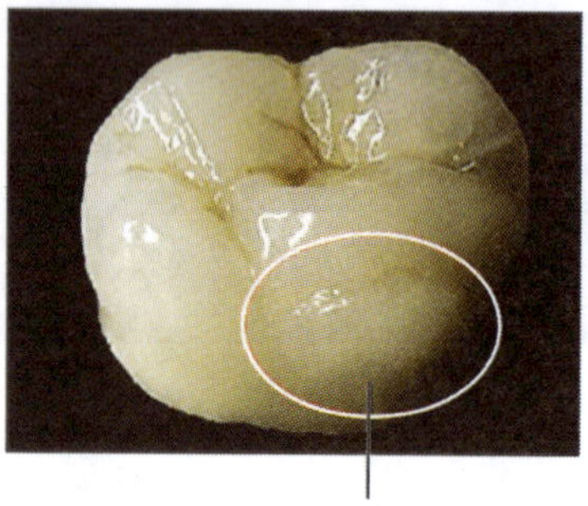
Carabelli cusp

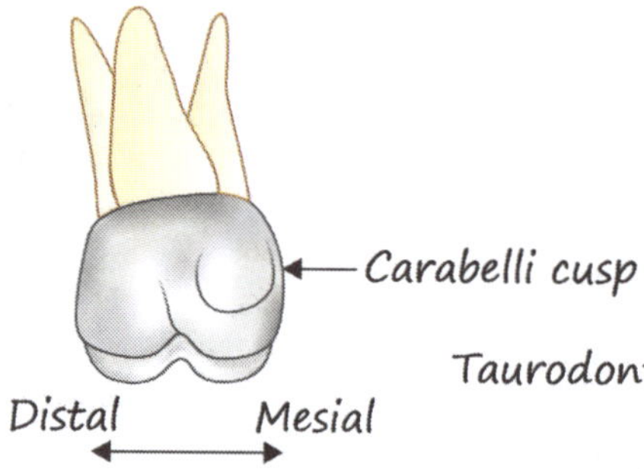

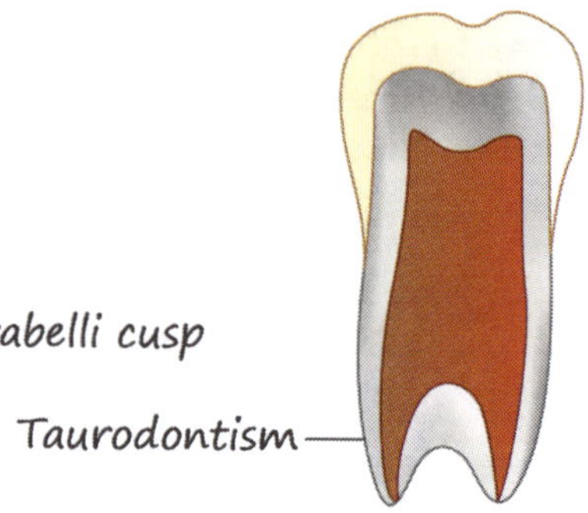

Mnemonic:

MONGOLOID TEETH

SET

S: Shovel incisors

E: Enamel pearl

T: Taurodontism

SEX DETERMINATION

Intersex:

- Intermingling of sexual characters of either sex in one individual[Q].
- Natural or acquired ('hijras' are castrated before puberty and 'zenanas[Q]' are castrated after puberty).

Concealed sex[Q]

- Individuals who hide their real sex by cross-dressing with a motive.
- Criminals may try to conceal their sex to avoid detection by the police, which can be identified by physical examination[Q].

DETERMINATION OF SEX FROM BONES

Sex Determination from Pelvis

Best suited[Q] for sex determination.

The **greater sciatic notch**[Q] is the *single most important differentiating feature*[Q] even in fetal life.

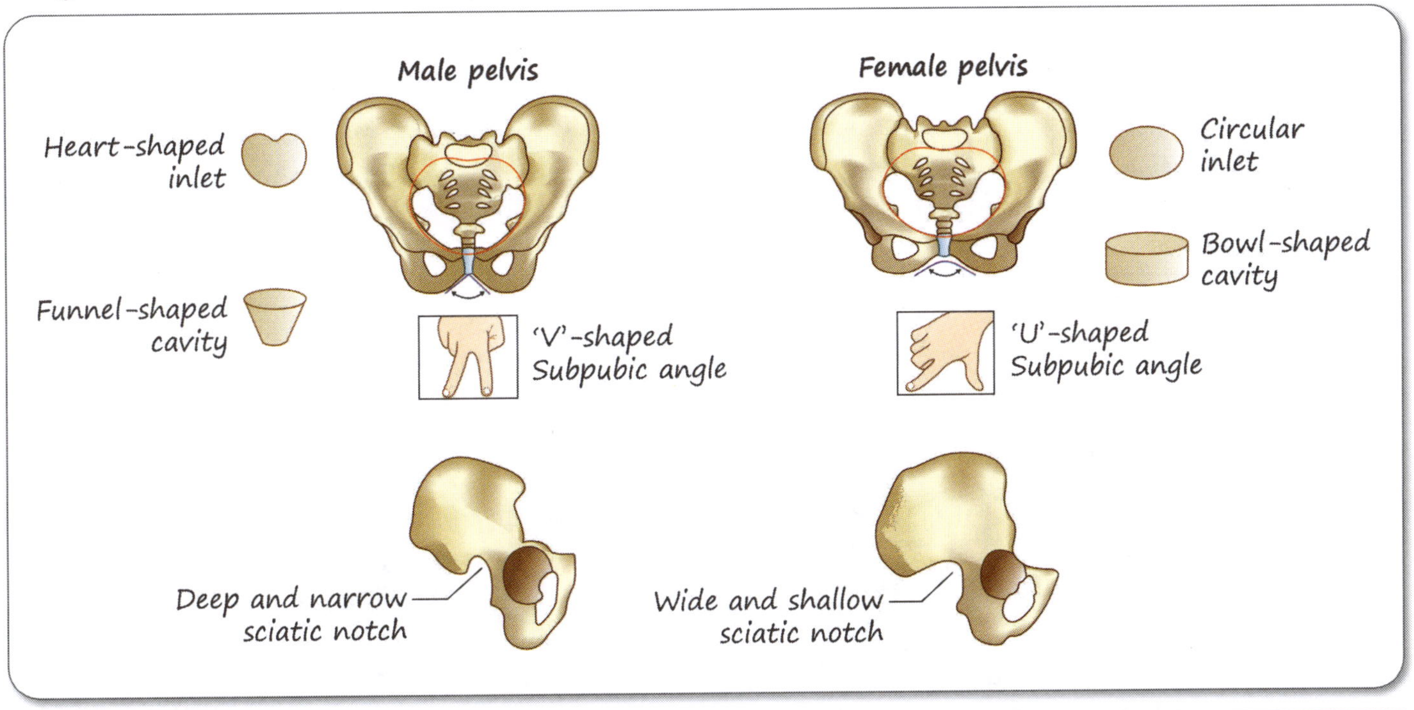

Feature	Male	Female
Pelvic inlet	Heart shaped	*Circular shaped*[Q]
Pelvic cavity	Funnel[Q]	Flat bowl
Preauricular sulcus	Narrow, shallow Not frequent	Broad[Q], deep more frequent[Q] (evidence of pregnancy)
Subpubic angle (SPA)	'v' shaped Acute (<90°)	'u' shaped obtuse[Q] (<90°)
Greater sciatic notch (75%)	*Narrower*[Q] *and deeper*	Wider[Q] and shallower
Obturator foramen	Large and oval	Small and triangular
Acetabulum	Large, directed laterally	Small, directed anterolaterally
Ischial tuberosity	Inverted	Everted

Contd...

Feature	Male	Female
Sacrum	Long Uniform curvature[Q] Promontory more prominent	Small Upper half straight, lower half curved forward. Promontory less prominent.
Pubis body	Triangular	Square

Sex Determination from Skull

Feature	Male	Female
Architecture	Rugged	Smooth
Muscle markings and bony ridges (glabella, supraorbital ridges, occipital protuberance, zygomatic arch, mastoid process)	More pronounced[Q]	Less pronounced
Frontal eminence and parietal eminence	Small	Large[Q]
Orbits	Square[Q] with smooth margin	Rounded with sharp margin
Fore head	Sloping and Steeper[Q]	Vertical
Palate	Large, broader and U-shaped	Smaller and parabola
Frontonasal junction	Distinct and angulated	Smooth
Diagastric groove	More deep	Less deep
Mastoid process	Large and blunt	Small and pointed

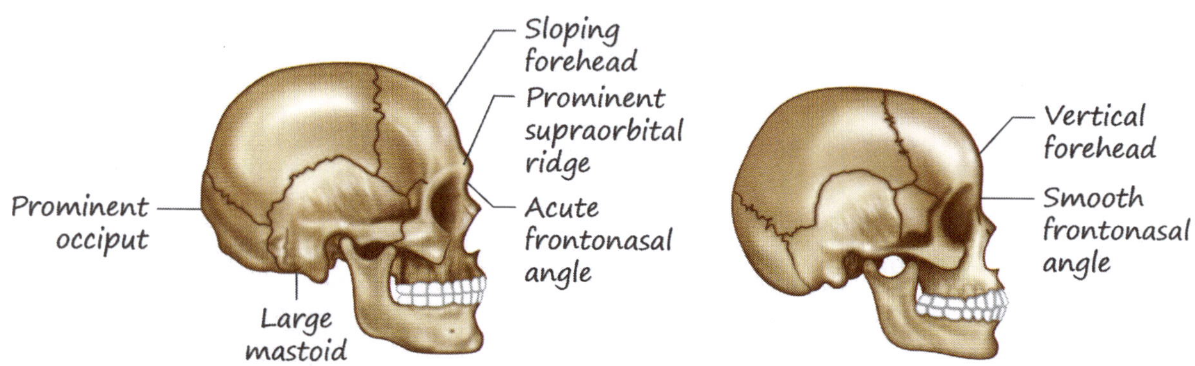

Sex Determination from Mandible

Feature	Male	Female
Appearance	**Large**—prominent muscle markings	**Small**—not prominent muscle markings
Chin	Square shaped[Q]	Rounded[Q]
Angle of body with ramus	Less obtuse <125°	More obtuse >125°
Angle of mandible	Everted[Q]	Inverted[Q]

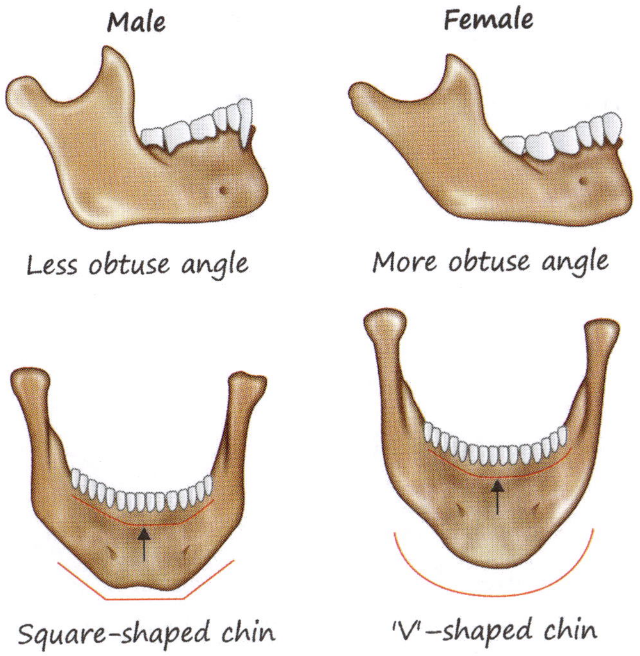

Krogman's accuracy[Q]: Diagnostic accuracy in sexing from bones

Recognizable sex differences in the bones appear *after puberty except* **in pelvis**[Q], where it is present since birth.

Krogman's accuracy

- Entire skeleton—100%
- Pelvis alone[Q]—95%
- Skull alone[Q]—92%
- Long bones—80%
- Pelvis + skull—98%
- Pelvis + Long bones—98%

Ashley's rule

- To determine the sex of the sternum.
- It's also known as '149 rule'.
- Male sternum length is >149 mm and female sternum length is <149 mm.

Indices for race

B—Brachial index
C—Crural index
C—Cephalic index
I—Intermembral index/intramembral index

Few indices for sex

Sleepy—Sternal index
Sarah—Sacral index
Slept—Sciatic index
In—Ischiopubic index
Class—Corporobasal index

All the indices are more in female except corporobasal index.
Best index to determine sex from pelvis is **Ischiopubic index**

AGE DETERMINATION

Age determination

- **Fetal age**
  Rule of Hasse/Morrison ossification centers
- **Before puberty**
  Teeth
  - Eruption
  - Mineralization (superior)
  - Boydes method
  - Stacks method

  Ossification centers
- **After puberty**
  Pubic symphyseal surface—Degenerative changes (best criteria)
  Skull suture closure
  Teeth—Secondary changes

Gestational Age Estimation from Crown to Heel Length

1st 5 months GA = $\sqrt{\text{Crown to heel length}}$ (Rule of Hasse)	2nd 5 months = CHL/5 = GA (Morrison's rule)

CRL = Crown to rump length

CRL = CHL × 2/3; CHL = CRL × 3/2

Clavicle (1st bone to ossify):

- Two primary ossification centers—6th Week of intrauterine life.
- Medial end of clavicle: Appearance by 18–19 years and fuses by 21–22 years.

Age Estimation from Ossification Centers of Wrist Joint and Carpal Bones

Wrist joint centers	Appearance	Fusion
Lower end of radius	2 years	18–19 years
Lower end of ulna	5–6 years	17–18 years
Capitate	2 months	
Hamate	3 months–1 year	
Triquetral	3 years	
Lunate	4 years	
Trapezium	5–6 years	
Trapezoid	5–6 years	
Scaphoid	5 years	
Pisiform	9–12 years	
Base of 1st	At birth	15 years

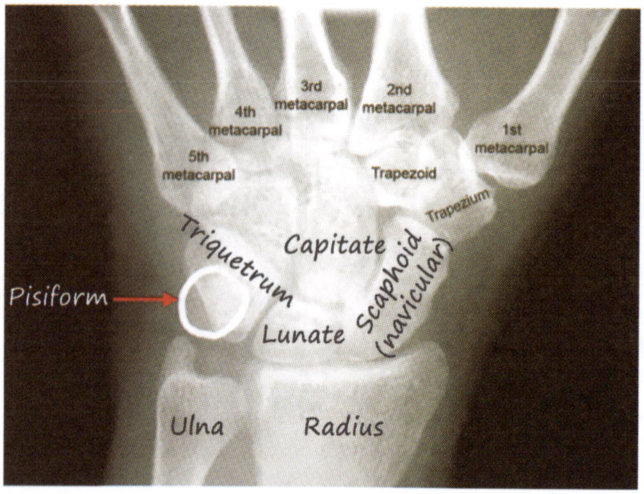

- **Two halves of mandible fuse together:** 1–2 years
- ***Basiocciput and basisphenoid: 18–21 years***[Q]

Sagittal suture	Coronal suture	Lambdoid suture
Posterior 1/3rd: 30–40 years	**Upper half:** 40–50 years	**Upper half:** 50–60 years
Anterior 1/3rd: 40–50 years	**Lower half:** 50–60 years	**Lower half:** 60–70 years
Middle 1/3rd: 50–60 years		

Age Estimation from Skull

- ***Closure of posterior fontanelle (Lambda***[Q]***):*** 3 months–6 months
- ***Closure of anterior fontanelle (Bregma***[Q]***):*** 1½–2 years[Q]
- ***Closure of metopic suture:*** 9 months–2 years

Certain facts regarding skull sutural closure

- **Reliability:** Sagittal suture > lambdoid > Coronal suture
- Endocranial suture closure occurs 5–10 years earlier than ectocranial suture.
- **Lapsed union**[Q]: Ectocranial suture may not close. (commonly seen in sagittal suture[Q].)

Age Estimation from Pelvis

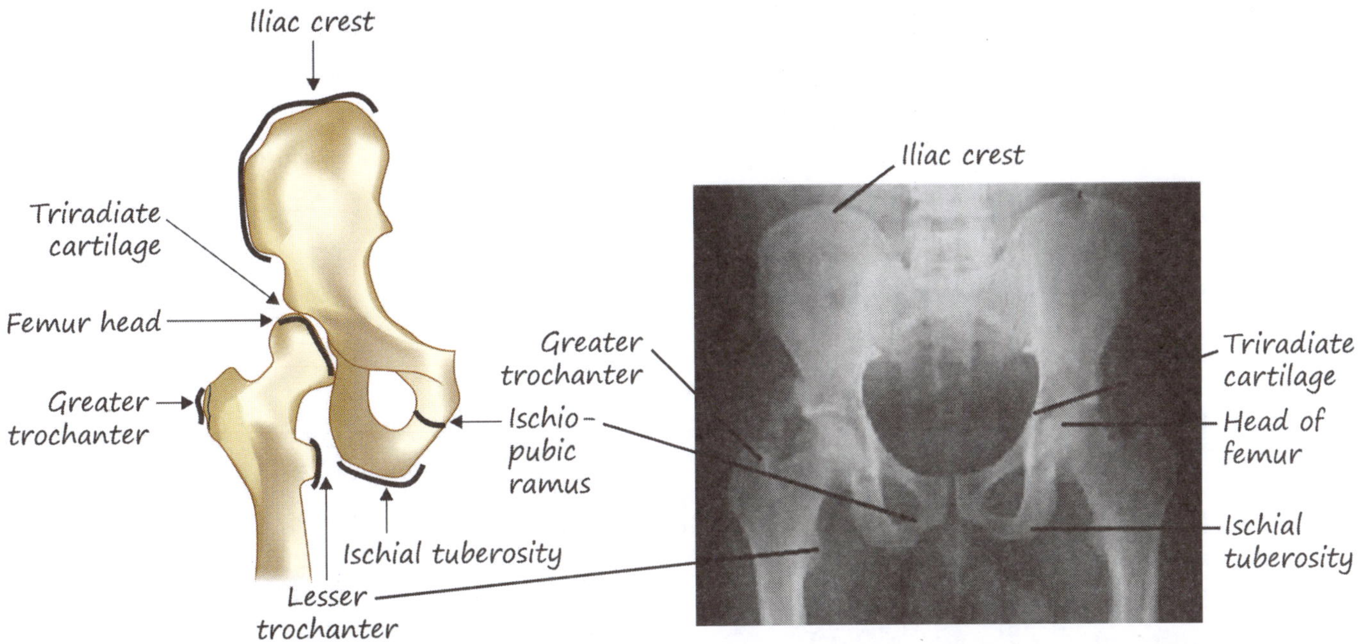

Pelvis ossification centers	Appearance	Fusion
Ischiopubic ramus		6th year
Triradiate cartilage		13–15 years
Ischial tuberosity	16 years	20–22 years
Iliac crest	14 years	18–20 years
Head of femur	1 year	17–18 years
Greater trochanter	4 years	17–18 years
Lesser trochanter	12–14 years	17–18 years

Age Estimation from Elbow Joint

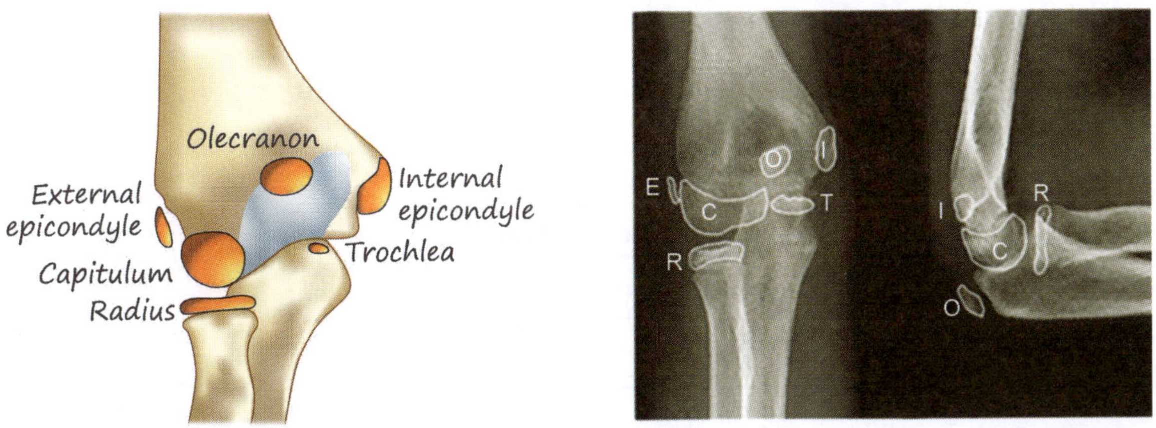

Mnemonic:

CRITOE	Elbow joint centers	Appearance	Fusion
C	Capitulum	1 year	16–17 years
R	Radial head	2 years	16–17 years
I	Inner (medial) epicondyle	5–7 years	16 years
T	Trochlea	9 years	16–17 years
O	Olecronon process of ulna	9 years	16–17 years
E	External lateral epicondyle	11 years	13 years

Sternum

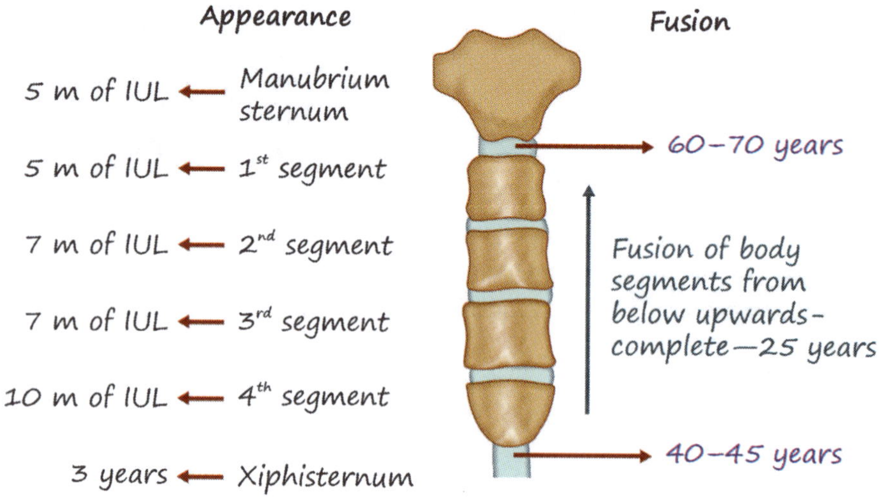

Sacrum Ossification

- The five sacral vertebrae remain separated until puberty and with the onset of puberty, ossification starts from below upwards and fusion becomes complete by 20–25 years.
- Sacrum becomes a single bone by 22–25 years.

Age Estimation from Teeth

Temporary dentition	Permanent dentition
• 20 teeth in number	• 32 teeth in number
• 2 incisors 1 canine 2 molars in each quadrant	• 2 incisors 1 canine 2 premolars 3 molars in each quadrant

Temporary dentition

Right upper quadrant					Left upper quadrant				
M2	M1	C	LI	CI	CI	LI	C	M1	M2
M2	M1	C	LI	CI	CI	LI	C	M1	M2
Right lower quadrant					Left lower quadrant				

Mnemonic:

Mnemonic	Temporary dentition	Average age of eruption (months)	Age in ranges (months)
I (incisors)	Lower central incisor (CI)	6	6–8
	Upper central incisor (CI)	7	7–9
	Upper lateral incisor (LI)	8	7–9
	Lower lateral incisor (LI)	9	10–12
Make	First molar (M1)	12	12–14
Chocolate	Canine (C)	18	17–19
Mousse	Second molar (M2)	24	20–30

Permanent dentition

Right upper quadrant								Left upper quadrant							
M3	M2	M1	PM2	PM1	C	LI	CI	CI	LI	C	PM1	PM2	M1	M2	M3
M3	M2	M1	PM2	PM1	C	LI	CI	CI	LI	C	PM1	PM2	M1	M2	M3
Right lower quadrant								**Left lower quadrant**							

Mnemonic:

Mnemonic	Permanent dentition	Average age of eruption (years)	Age (years)
Mummy	First molar (MI)	6	6–7
	(First to erupt)		
Is	Central incisor (CI)	7	6–8
In	Lateral incisor (LI)	8	7–9
Pain	First premolar (PM1)	9	9–11
Papa	Second premolar (PM2)	10	10–12
Can	Canine (C)	11	11–12
Make	Second molar (M2)	12	12–14
Medicine	Third molar (M3)	17–25	17–25
	(Last to erupt)		

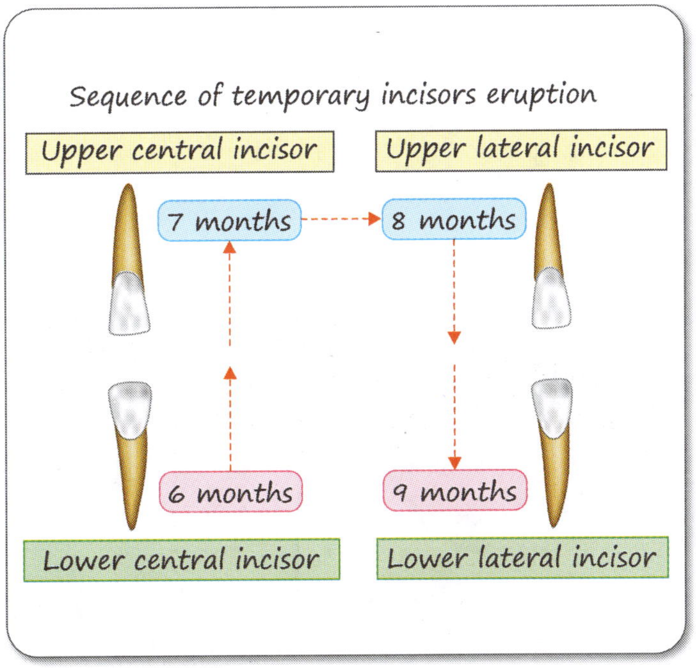

Rule of Half Dozen: Multiples of 6

Eruption sequence of temporary teeth

- Incisors: 6 months
- 1st molar: 12 months
- Canine: 18 months
- 2nd molar: 24 months

Period of Mixed Dentition: (6–11 years)

Both the **temporary teeth and permanent teeth present in the oral cavity** between **6 years and 11 years**

Superadded teeth
Teeth which don't have deciduous predecessors All *permanent molars*[Q] 12 in number[Q]
Successional teeth
Teeth which erupt in the place of deciduous teeth Permanent incisors, canines and premolars 20 in numbers[Q]

Chronological Sequence of Permanent Dentition Eruption

Age	Erupting teeth	Total number of teeth in the oral cavity
6 years[Q]	Permanent 1st molar *(first)*[Q]	24[Q] (4 P + 20 T)[Q]
7 years	Permanent central incisors	24[Q] (8 P + 16 T)
8 years	Permanent lateral incisors	24[Q] (12 T and 12 P)[Q]
9 years	Permanent 1st premolar	24[Q] (8 T and 16 P)[Q]
10 years	Permanent 2nd premolar	24[Q] (4 T and 20 P)
11 years	Permanent canine	24[Q]
12 years	Permanent 2nd molar	28
17–25 years	Permanent 3rd molar *(last)*[Q]	32

Formula to calculate total number of permanent teeth in oral cavity from age
No. of permanent teeth = (Age in years – 5) × 4

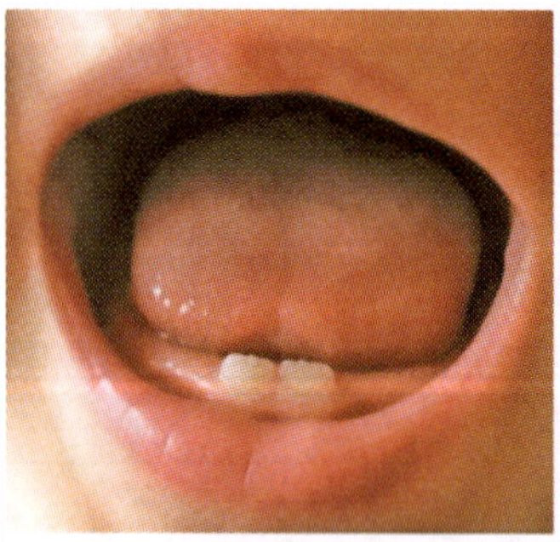

First temporary tooth to erupt—lower central incisor

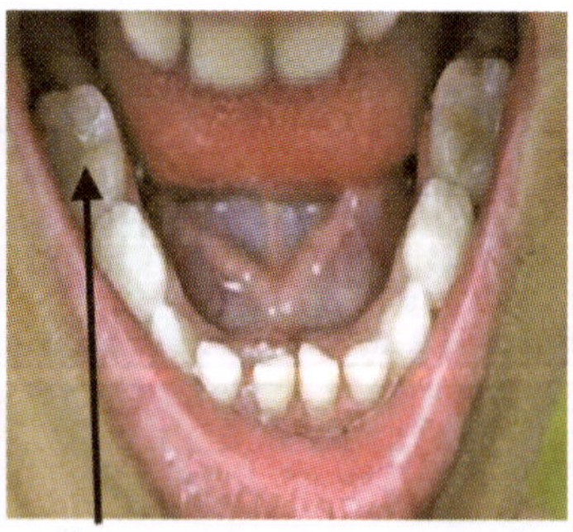

First permanent tooth to erupt—molar 1

Other Methods of Age Estimation from Teeth

Boyde's method (based on incremental growth lines[Q] in tooth)	Stack's method
• Neonatal line appears in about 3 days (electron microscope) to 3 weeks (simple microscope). • Age is calculated by counting the number of lines from the neonatal line[Q]. • Useful to estimate the age of a dead infant. • Age can be determined in terms of days[Q].	• Age is estimated from the height and weight of the erupting tooth[Q]. • Used in fetus and infants[Q]

Gustafson's Method (Based on Secondary Changes in Teeth)

Criteria	Mnemonic APSRTC
1. Attrition[Q]: Wear and tear seen over the occlusal surface.	A: Attrition
2. Paradentosis: The gum margins become retracted and there is loosening of teeth.	P: Paradentosis
3. **Secondary dentin[Q]: (Second most reliable criteria)** Deposition of dentin (secondarily) within the pulp cavity.	S: Secondary dentin[Q]
4. **Root resorption:** Root resorption due to aging.	R: Root resorption
5. **Transparency of root[Q]: (most reliable criteria)** Transparency of the dentin at the root level.	T: Transparency of root[Q]
6. **Cementum apposition:** Apposition of cementum at and around the root of the teeth.	C: Cementum deposition

- Anterior to posterior teeth: reliability decreases (**Incisors more reliable[Q]** > molars not reliable)
- ***Attrition and paradentosis are the only criteria useful for living persons.***

Lamendin Method

Age estimation from gum recession and transparency of root

DENTAL CHARTING METHODS

Universal (Cunningham) System (permanent teeth are numbered from 1 to 32; Deciduous teeth are lettered from A to T)

In a clockwise direction.

Palmer's Notation[Q] (Adult teeth are numbered 1–8; Deciduous teeth are indicated by a letter A to E)

The Palmer notation consists of a symbol (┘└┐┌) designating in which quadrant the tooth is found and a number indicating the position from the midline.

Palmer notation

Permanent teeth															
Upper right								Upper left							
8┘	7┘	6┘	5┘	4┘	3┘	2┘	1┘	└1	└2	└3	└4	└5	└6	└7	└8
8┐	7┐	6┐	5┐	4┐	3┐	2┐	1┐	┌1	┌2	┌3	┌4	┌5	┌6	┌7	┌8
Lower right								Lower left							

Deciduous teeth															
Upper right								Upper left							
			E┘	D┘	C┘	B┘	└A	└A	└B	└C	└D	└E			
			E┐	D┐	C┐	B┐	┌A	┌A	┌B	┌C	┌D	┌E			
Lower right								Lower left							

Haderup System[Q]

- This is a method of eight tooth quadrant system in which plus (+) and minus (−) were used to differentiate between upper and lower quadrants.
- For right quadrants, Plus sign is used on the right side of tooth number; For left quadrants, plus sign is used on the left side of the tooth number. (e.g., +1 = upper right central incisor; 1− = lower left central incisor).

Federation Dentaire Internationale (FDI) System

- Internationally adopted system[Q]
- Each tooth is identified by a two-digit number in which, **the proximal digit indicates the quadrant[Q] and the distal digit indicates the actual tooth[Q].**

Prefix number:

- **Permanent teeth:** 1, 2, 3, 4 are used for designating right upper, left upper, left lower and right lower quadrants respectively.
- **Temporary teeth:** 5,6,7,8 are used for the corresponding temporary teeth.

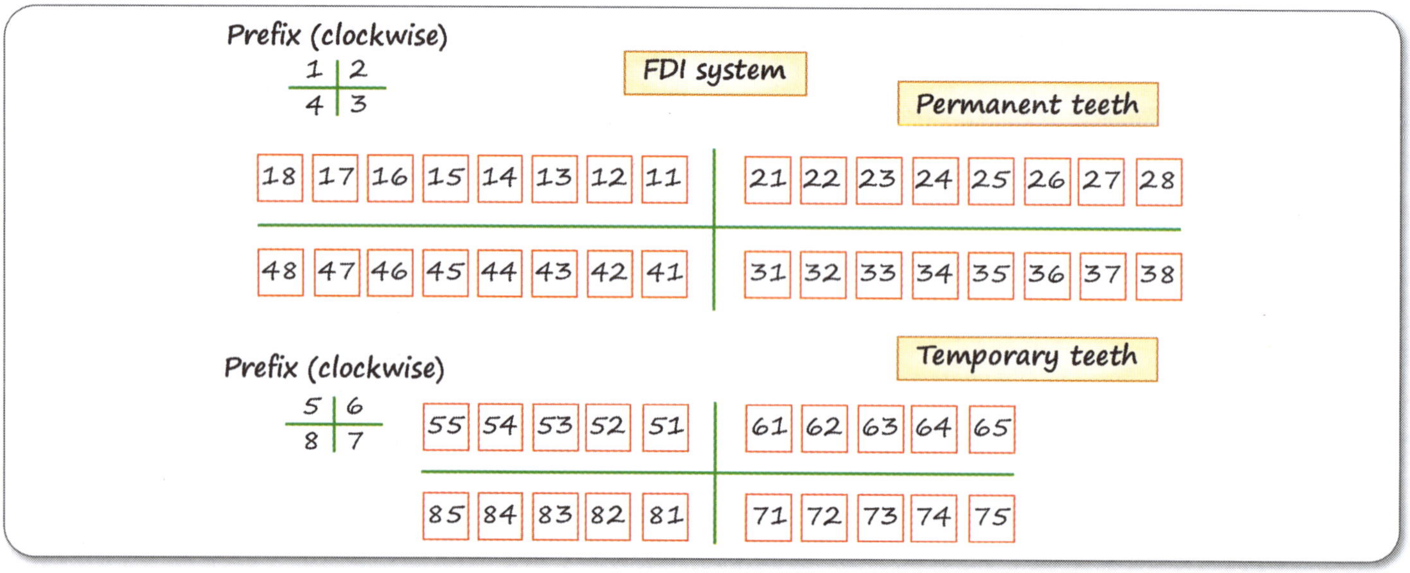

MEDICOLEGAL IMPORTANCE OF AGE

Chronological age	Medicolegal significance
4 months IUL	Sex[Q] can be recognized
7 months IUL	Viability[Q]
1 year	Infanticide (killing of an infant—punishable under 302 IPC)
<7 years[Q]	Not criminally responsible according to Sec. 82 IPC.
7–12 years	Criminally responsible if sufficient maturity present (Sec. 83 IPC[Q])
12 years	• Minimum age to give consent for physical examination[Q]. ▪ Consent given by child <12 years is invalid (90 IPC) ▪ In such cases, Consent of the guardian is required (89 IPC) • Minimum age to take oath[Q]. • Exposure and abandonment of child <12 years by parent is punishable (317 IPC)
<14 years	Cannot be employed in factory jobs
14–15 years	Nonhazardous jobs in factories can be given

Contd...

Chronological age	Medicolegal significance
<16 years	Taking away a male without the consent of the guardian is kidnapping Punishable under 363 IPC
>18 years **Mnemonic:** ADOLESCENT	• Taking away a girl from lawful guardian amounts to kidnapping. A : Attainment of majority/age of marriage for girls. DO : Donation of organs. L : Licence (driving). E : Election (elligible to vote). S : Sexual intercourse consent. C : Consent for major procedures, MTP. EN : Employment (Naukri). T : Testamentary capacity (eligible to write a valid will).
21 years	• Majority[Q] (when the individual is under guardianship of court) • Marriage age for boys • Procuring a female from abroad for prostitution is punishable.
>25 years	Minimum age for a MP
35 years	Minimum age for president, VP, and Governor

DACTYLOGRAPHY—FINGERPRINTING STUDY

- Fingerprints are the impressions of the papillary ridges on the skin/surface.
- First used in India by Sir William Herschel (1858) and first systematized by Sir Francis Galton[Q] (1892)
- First fingerprint bureau of the world was established at Calcutta[Q] (1897)
- In practice **12–16 points of comparison**[Q] are accepted as proof of identity.
- Development of fingerprint starts 12–16 weeks of IUL (3–4 months) and fingerprint completion occurs by 20–24 weeks of IUL (5–6 months).

Advantages of fingerprints

- Most reliable method of identification[Q].
- Absolutely individualistic (Chance of two individuals having same fingerprints is 1 in 64 billion)
- Different even in identical twins[Q].
- Not inherited[Q]. (not used for paternity tesing)

Mnemonic:

Types of fingerprints pattern: CLAW

C : Composite;
L : Loops;
A : Arch;
W : Whorls

Types (as recovered in crime scene):

1. Visible/patent/chance: Blood stained prints
2. Invisible/latent: Needs development techniques to make it visible.
3. Plastic/indented: Fingerprint gets embedded when finger touches molten surface.

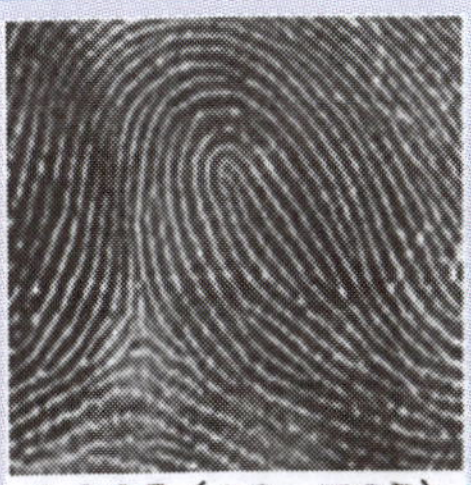

LOOP (60–70%) (most commonQ)

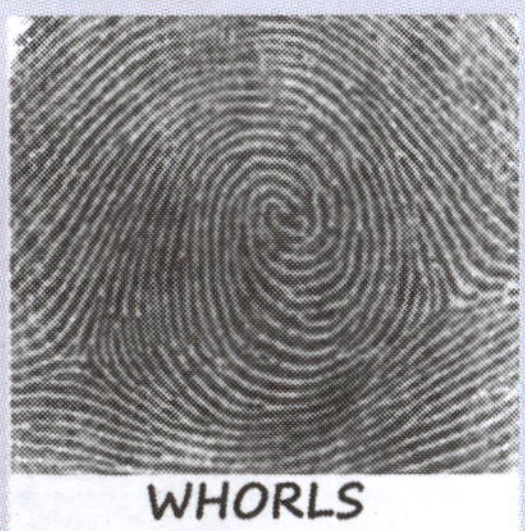

WHORLS (25–35%)

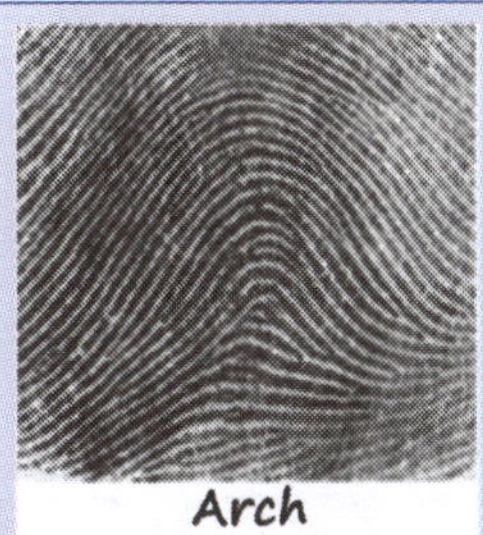

Arch (6–7%)

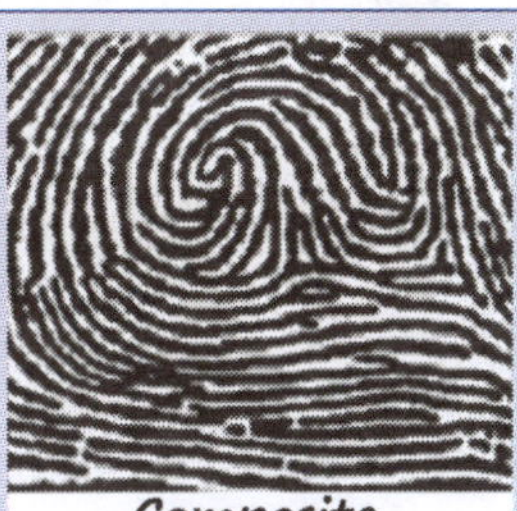

Composite (1–2%)

Extra Edges

Modifications of Fingerprint Pattern

PERMANENT ALTERATION OF FINGERPRINT PATTERN	
• Leprosy[Q]	• Electrocution[Q]
• Radiation exposure	• Skin grafting

INCREASE DISTANCE BETWEEN RIDGES
• Acromegaly
• Infantile paralysis
• Rickets

RIDGE ATROPHY	
Complete atrophy	**Incomplete Atrophy**
Coeliac disease	Dermatitis

Poroscopy

- Poroscopy is the study of pore structures[Q] found on the papillary ridges of the fingers for identification.
- Developed by Edmund Locard[Q].

Principle:

- Fingerprint ridges are studded with microscopic pores, which are the **openings of sweat glands[Q]**.
- Each millimeter of ridge contains 9–18 pores.
- The characteristics of pores are **unique to each individual and permanent[Q]**.

Locard's poroscopy

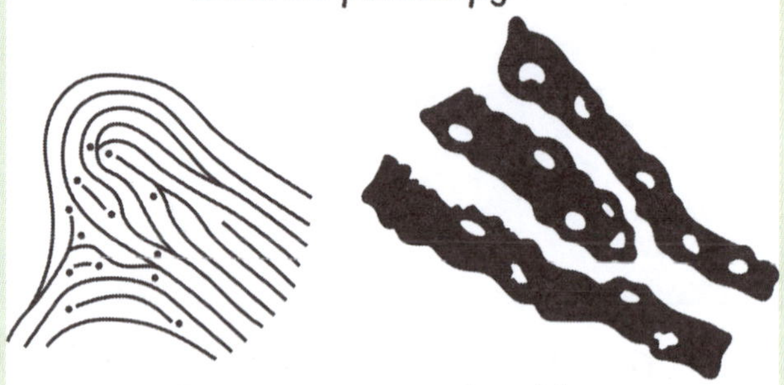

Sweat pores on the ridges

Suzuki Classification

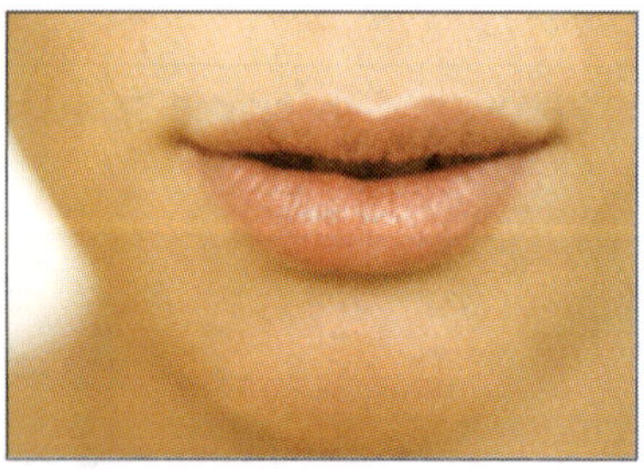

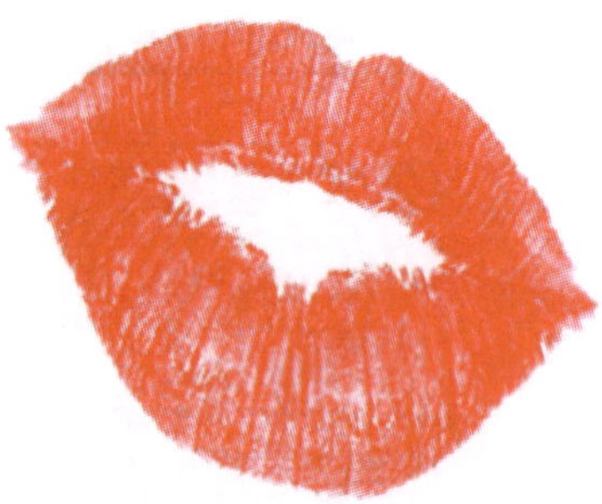

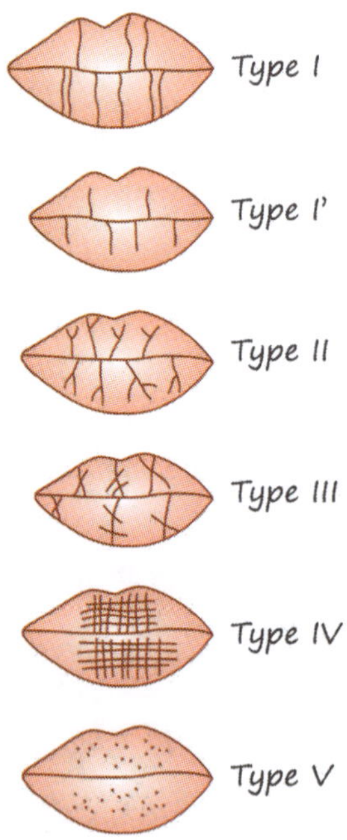

Lip Prints (Cheiloscopy)

- **Cheiloscopy[Q]** is the study of **lip prints**.
- Lip prints are unique and used for **personal identification**.
- Found in the objects at the scene of crime, e.g., cutlery and crockery items, cigarette ends, etc.

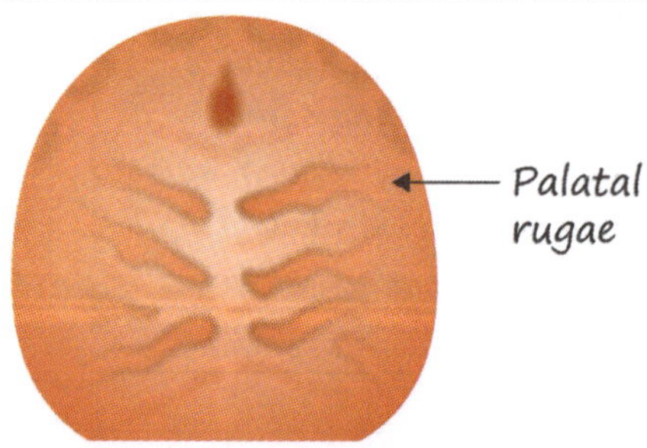

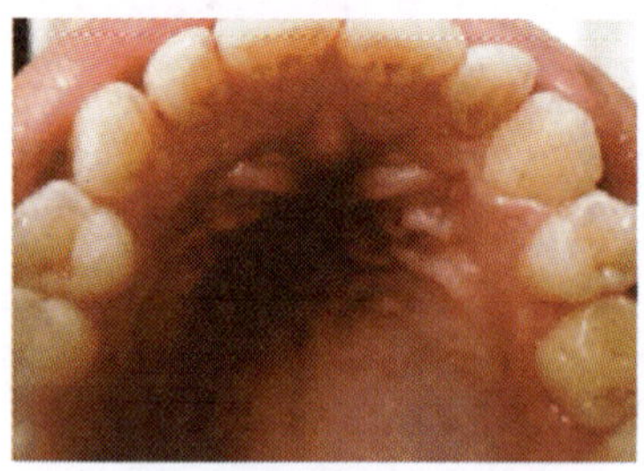

Palatoscopy/Palato-Print/Rugoscopy

The **study of palatal rugae**[Q] in the **hard palate**[Q] to establish identity.

Principle: Rugae pattern remains stable throughout life and does not change during growth.

Location: Anterior third of the palate[Q], behind the incisive papilla.

- Three types of rugae: Primary rugae (>5 mm); secondary rugae (3–5 mm) and tertiary rugae (<3 mm)
- Palatine rugae are unique and can be used for identification.
- Can be used even in advanced decomposition.
- Rugae are protected from trauma due to its situation and from heat by buccal pad of fat and tongue.

Tattoo Marks

- Tattoo marks are designs produced by multiple punctures of skin with needles dipped in pigments.
- Common dyes used: Indian ink, indigp, Prussian blue, vermillion.
- Faint or disappeared tattoo marks can be made out on histological study of the **regional lymph nodes**[Q].
- Drug addicts often imprint tattoos over areas of multiple injection mark, in order to conceal the needle puncture marks.

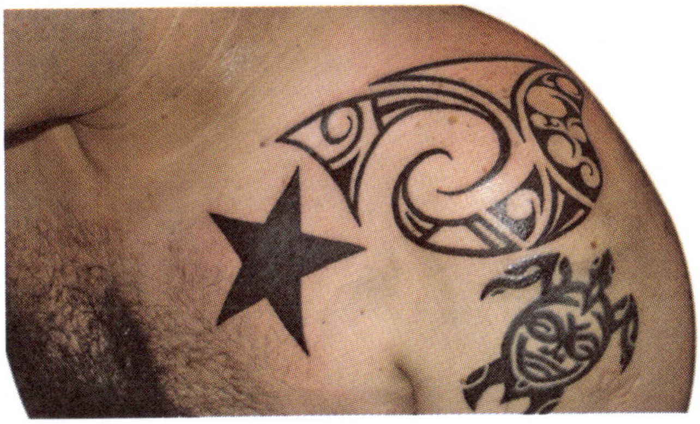

Tatoo mark

Methods to Demonstrate Old or Faint Tattoos

- **Infrared photography**[Q]
- **UV lamp**[Q]
- Magnifying glass
- High contrast photography

SUPERIMPOSITION TECHNIQUE

- Superimposition technique involves superimposing an image of the recovered skull over an ante mortem image of the suspected individual
- It determines whether the **skull belongs to the person in the photograph or not**[Q]

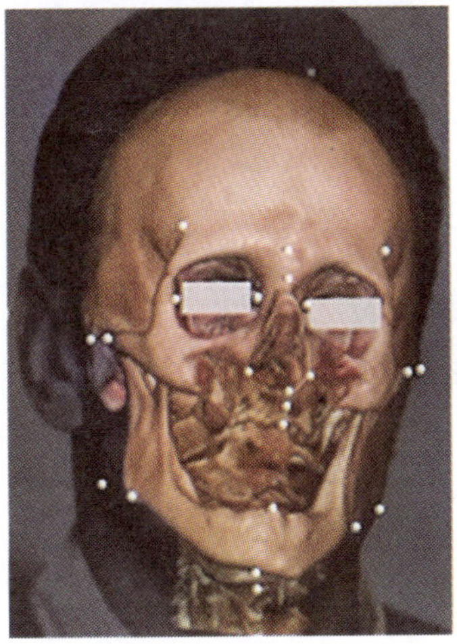

Superimposition technique

Method

- An unknown skull and a photo of the missing person are required for superimposition.
- The photograph is enlarged to natural size from the presence of some standard thing in the photograph of the missing person to indicate the scale. Comparison using landmarks is made.
- The resulting superimposed photograph brings out the points of similarity or dissimilarity between the photograph and the skull.
- Negative results are more significant[Q] rather than a positive match.

Transfer of evidences

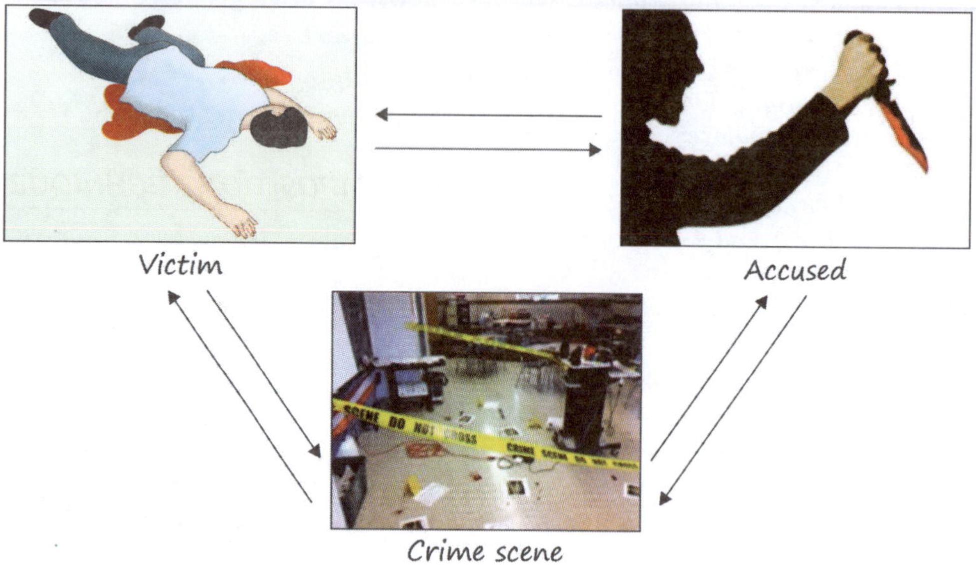

DETERMINATION OF STATURE

- Stature can be determined from skeletal bones by formulae (Karl Pearson's and Trotter and Glesser's) and multiplication factors
- Usually long bones are ideal for determining stature.
- Femur is the best bone used for stature estimation. Femur forms 27% of the entire stature of a person.

Percentage of stature contributed by bones
- Femur: 27%
- Tibia: 22%
- Humerus: 20%
- Spinal column: 35%

Multiplication factor for stature determination
- Femur: **3.7**
- Tibia and fibula: (3.7 + 0.8) = **4.5**
- Humerus: (4.5 + 0.8) = **5.3**
- Ulna: (5.3 + 0.8) = **6.1**
- Radius: **6.5**

3. ASPHYXIAL DEATHS

ASPHYXIA

- Asphyxia literally means pulselessness[Q].
- A condition caused by interference with the exchange of oxygen and carbon dioxide in the body.

Classical Signs of Asphyxia (Asphyxia Triad)

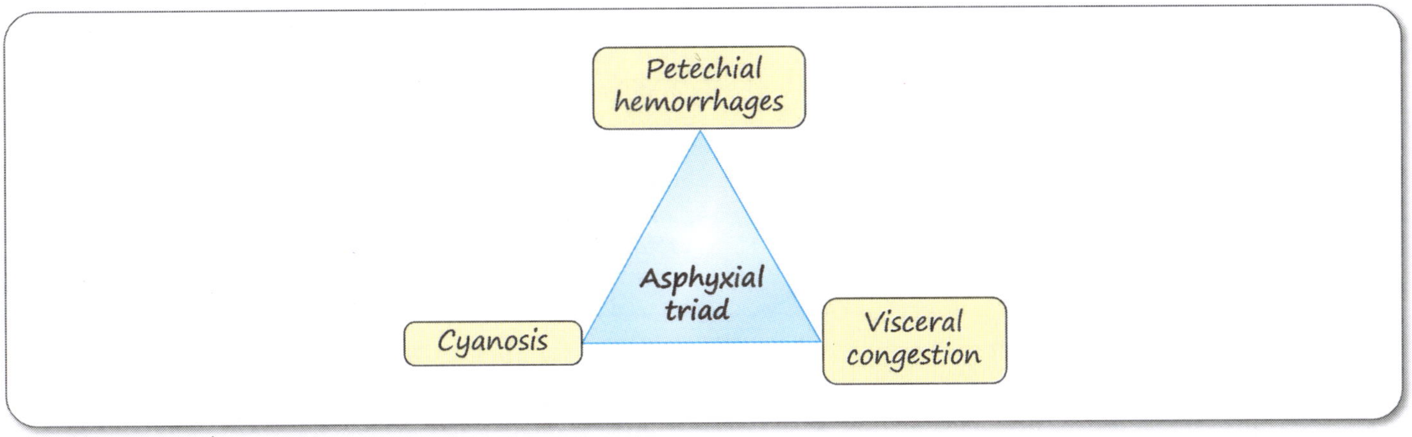

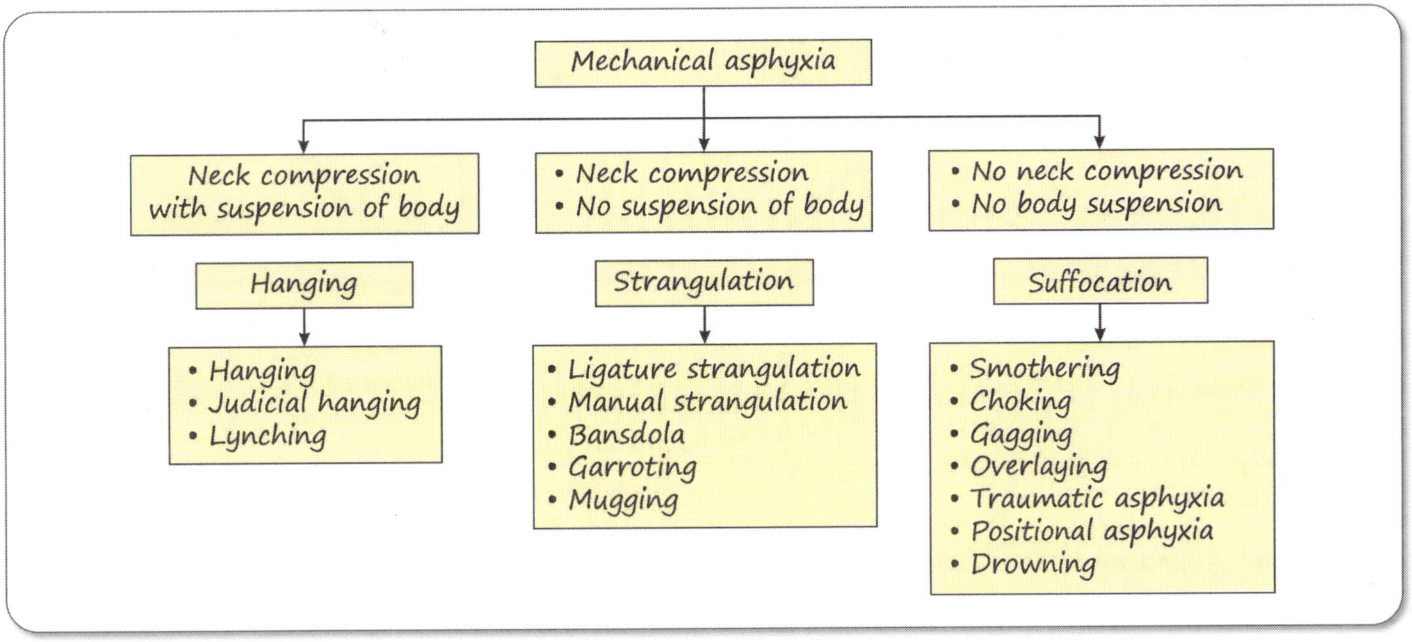

HANGING

- Hanging is a form of asphyxia caused by **suspension of the body** by a **ligature encircling the neck.**
- *The constricting force being the weight of the body*[Q]

Types of Hanging

- **Hanging**
  - Based on position of knot
    - **Typical hanging**
      - Knot is at occiput
      - Point of suspension is placed centrally
    - **Atypical hanging**
      - Knot of ligature is anywhere other than on the occiput
  - Based on degree of suspension
    - **Complete hanging**
      - Body is fully suspended
      - No body part touches the ground
      - Constricting force is weight of the body
    - **Partial hanging**
      - Any part of the body is touching the ground
      - For example, Sitting, kneeling, lying position
      - Weight of the head is the constricting force

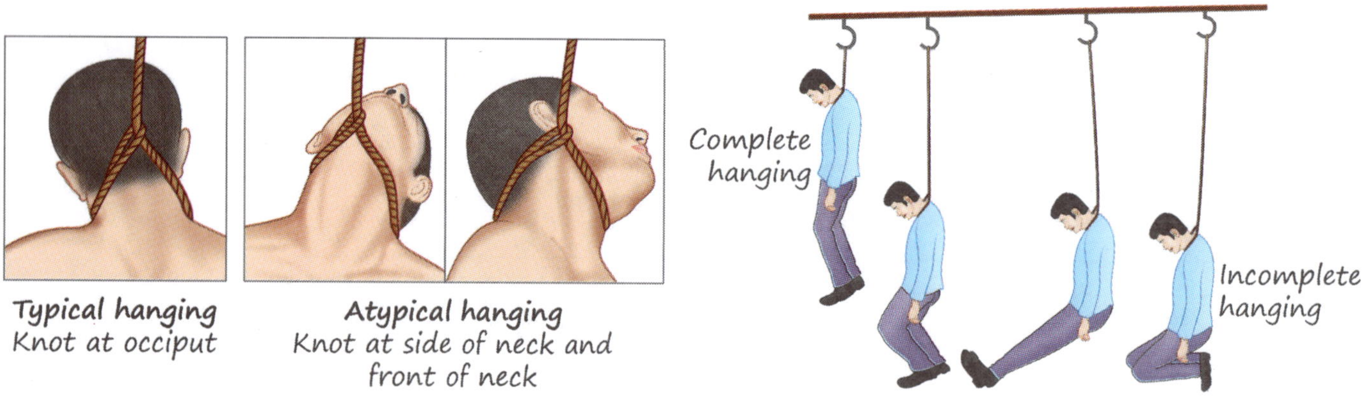

Fatal period: 3–5 minutes

Death is *immediate,* if cervical vertebrae are fractured (as in judicial hanging[Q]) or if the heart is inhibited, rapid if cause is asphyxia and *least rapid* if coma is responsible.

Postmortem Appearances in a Case of Hanging

External Findings

- Glove and stocking pattern hypostasis (in the lower part of legs and hands).
- Involuntary discharge of fecal matter and urine may be seen.
- In males, there may be penile erection and *involuntary discharge of semen*[Q].

Signs on Face

- **Tardieu's spots:** Over the eyelids, under the conjunctiva and near the temple.
- Cyanosis of face and subconjunctival hemorrhages and bleeding from nose/ears.
- Protrusion of tongue[Q] due to pressure on floor
- **La facie sympathique**[Q]
- Dribbling of saliva[Q]

Dribbling of saliva: *(Surest sign of antemortem hanging[Q])*

Pressure on submandibular salivary gland/pterygopalatine ganglion
↓
Stimulation of salivary gland
↓
Excessive salivary secretion
↓
Dribbling of saliva

Dribbling of saliva occurs from angle opposite to the side of the knot.
(When the knot is on the nape of the neck, it occurs across the middle of lower lip)

LE FACIE SYMPATHIQUE (originally described by Etienne Martin (1950))

- Sign of antemortem hanging[Q].
- *If the knot/ligature presses on cervical sympathetic chain[Q], eyelid of the that side remains open and the pupil is dilated[Q].*

Signs on Neck

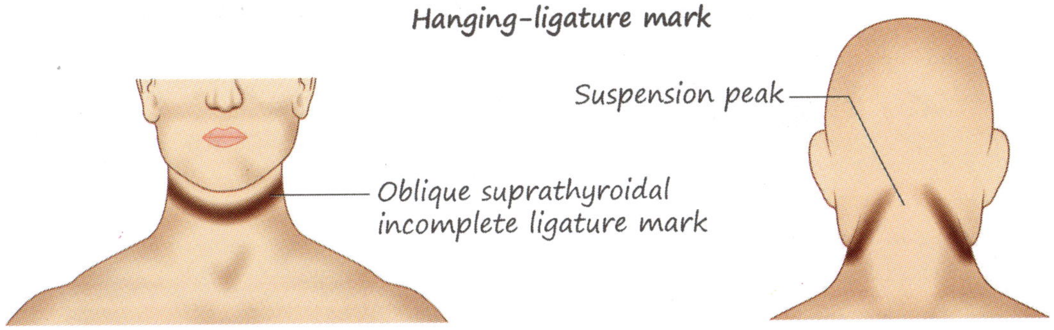

Ligature Mark (Suprathyroidal[Q], Oblique[Q], Incomplete[Q])

- Pressure abrasion[Q] (sometimes patterned—Patterned abrasion[Q]).
- Above the thyroid cartilage (usually).
- It runs obliquely, discontinuous, backward, upward and toward the point of suspension.
- *Mark is discontinuous[Q]* because of a gap produced by the knot at the nape of neck (**suspension peak**).
- Skin at the site: Usually **pale in color, but later becomes yellowish, dry and parchment like[Q]**.

- Transverse ligature mark is seen in:
    - Partial hanging
    - Low point of suspension
    - Slip knot with running noose

- Soft ligature causes wide/faint ligature mark.
- Narrow wire causes deep ligature mark (cheese cutters method).

Knots

Fixed knot: Oblique ligature mark and incomplete ligature mark.

Slip knot with running noose: Transverse and complete ligature mark.

Internal Findings

Neck

Subcutaneous tissue underneath the ligature mark is dry, white, firm and glistening[Q].

Hyoid bone fracture (15–20%)
- More commonly >40 year[Q]
- Abduction fracture[Q] or anterior compression fracture is seen
- Most common site[Q]: Junction of the inner two-thirds and outer-third of greater cornu

Amussat's sign[Q]
- Transverse carotid intimal tears[Q]
- Especially seen in long drops (judicial hanging[Q])

Fracture of vertebra
- Fracture of C2 vertebra (axis)—Hangman's fracture
- Fracture of pedicles or pars interarticularis of the axis vertebra (C2)
- Also resulting in spondylolisthesis of C2 over C3[Q]
- Associated with hyperextension of neck
- Also seen in sports, RTAs etc.

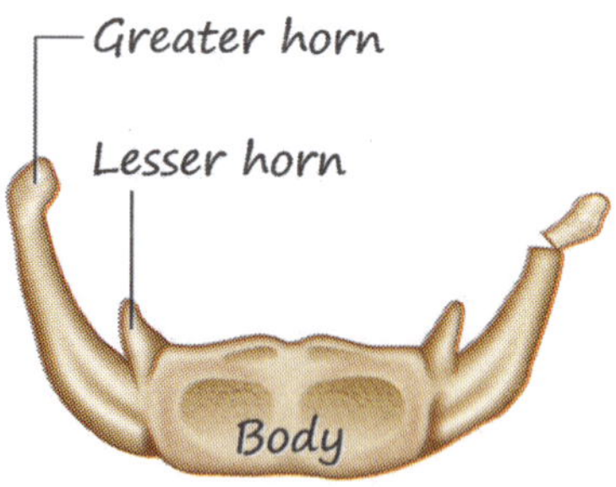

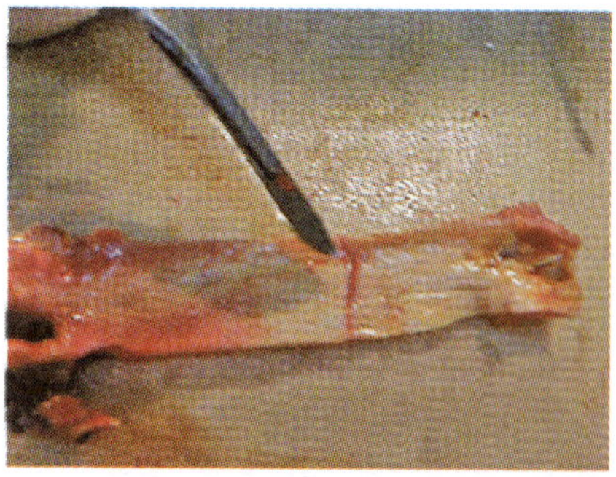

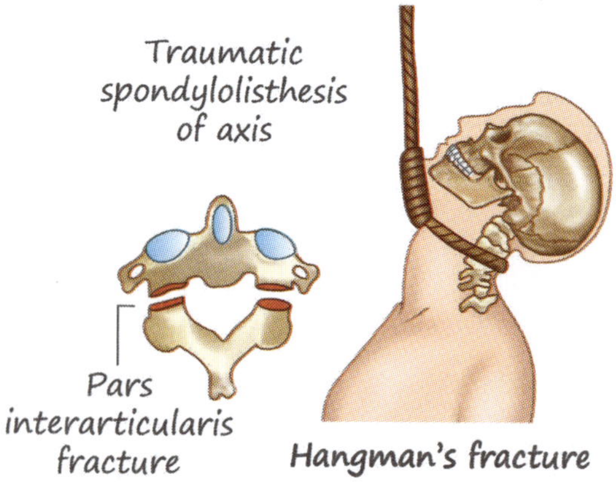

Hangman's fracture

Extra Edge

Simon's sign:
- **Stripe like** Hemorrhages seen on ventral surface of the intervertebral disks[Q] in lumbar vertebra.
- Due to overstretching of spine.
- **False positive:** Putrefaction, drowning and RTA

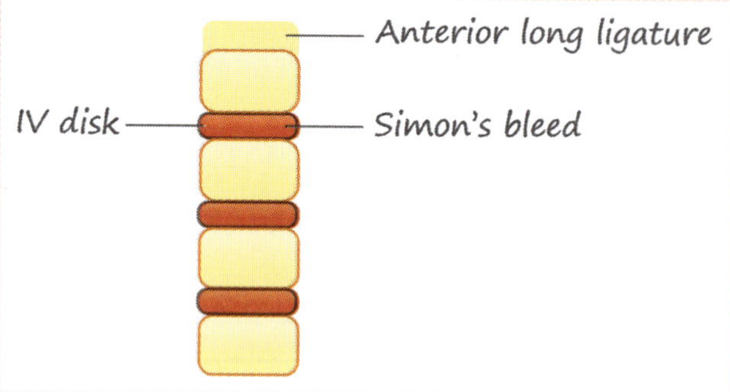

Suspension peak:
- The ligature mark of hanging is **incomplete at the position of the knot.**
- The gap resembles a **triangle with the apex upward.**
- This is called **suspension peak.**
- Indicates the position of the junction of the vertical part of the rope and the noose.

Importance:
It distinguishes hanging from ligature strangulation.

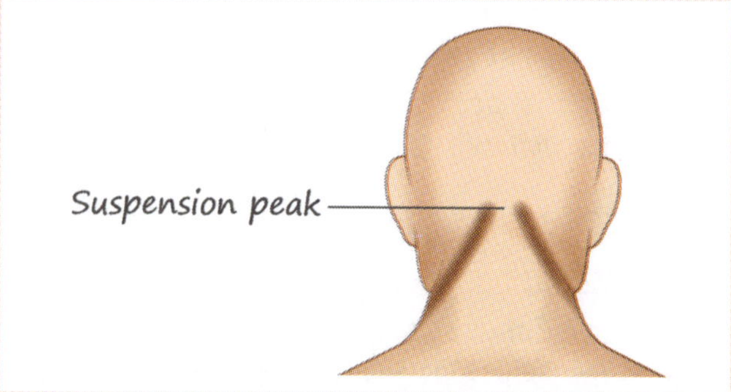

MANNER OF HANGING

Suicidal hanging
- Hanging is a common method of committing suicide, as it causes painless death
- Suicidal note[Q] may be present
- Fibers of the ligature material used, may be present in the hands

Homicidal hanging
- Very rare.

Homicide should be suspected, when:
- Signs of violence in the scene
- Injuries present

Accidental hanging
- Common in children, while 'playing hanging' or getting suspended from play equipment
- Autoerotic hanging[Q] in adults

LYNCHING

- Lynching is a form of **homicidal hanging**[Q].
- Extrajudicial Homicidal hanging by a mob in a public place.
- It was practiced by Captain William Lynch in North America, where the blacks accused of rape, were hanged publicly without any trial.

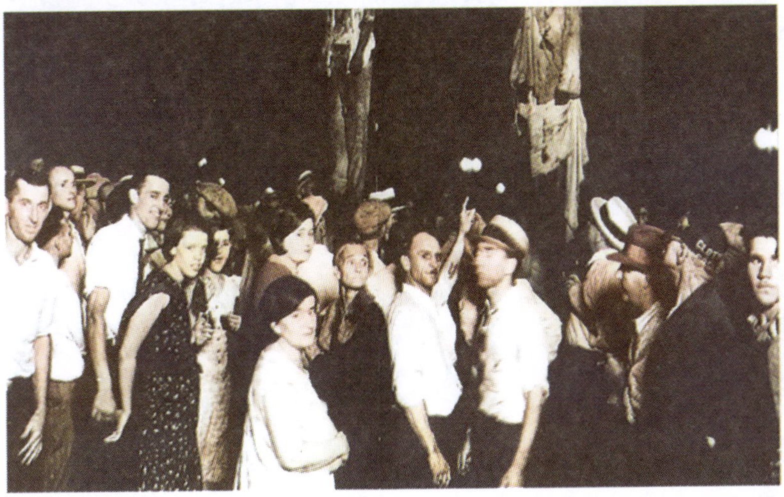

Lynching—Homicidal hanging by mob

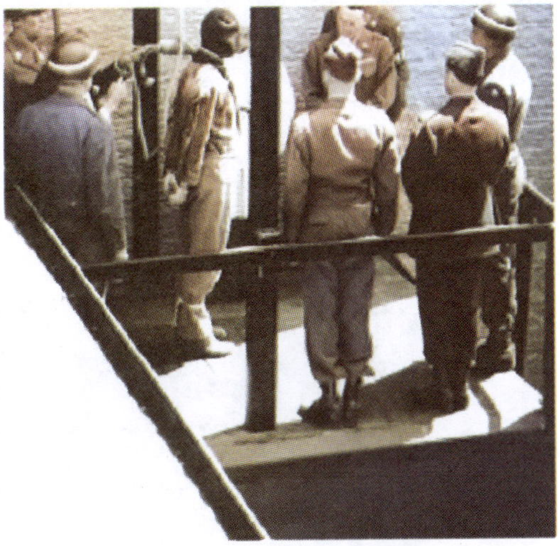

Judicial hanging

JUDICIAL HANGING

- **Hangman's knot:** Submental position (more effective).
- **In India, Knot:** Under the angle of jaw[Q].
- The ligature around the neck causes a forceful jerky impact on the neck and results in *Hangman's fracture*.

SEXUAL ASPHYXIA/AUTOEROTIC ASPHYXIA/HYPOXYPHILIA/ASPHYXIOPHILIA/KOCWARISM

Autoerotic asphyxia is a paraphilia in which sexual arousal and orgasm depend on self-induced asphyxia.

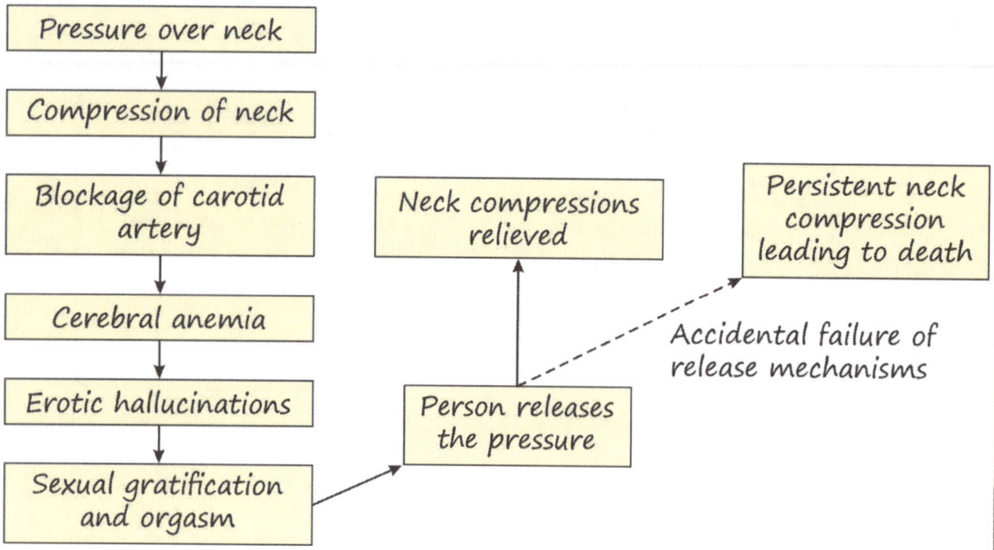

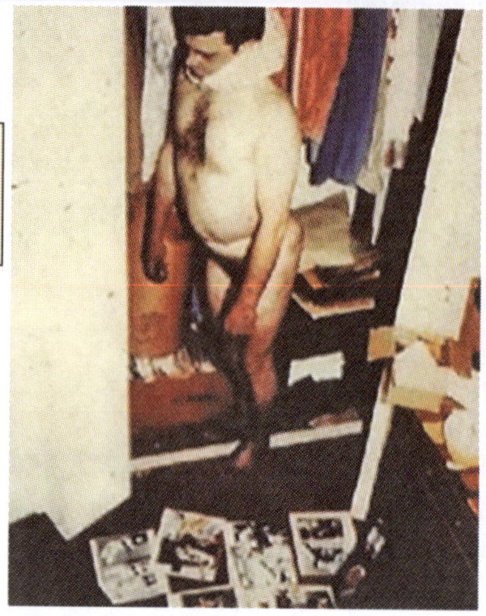

Methods

- Hanging^Q: Most frequent method.
- Electrical stimulation.
- A form of masochism. Transvestism is noted sometimes.

Scene is usually the victim's own house, bedroom, bathroom

- No disturbance^Q in the scene of crime
- Manner of death is accidental^Q.
- No suicidal note **present**^Q.

LIGATURE STRANGULATION

Ligature Strangulation (When Ligature Material is used to Constrict Neck)

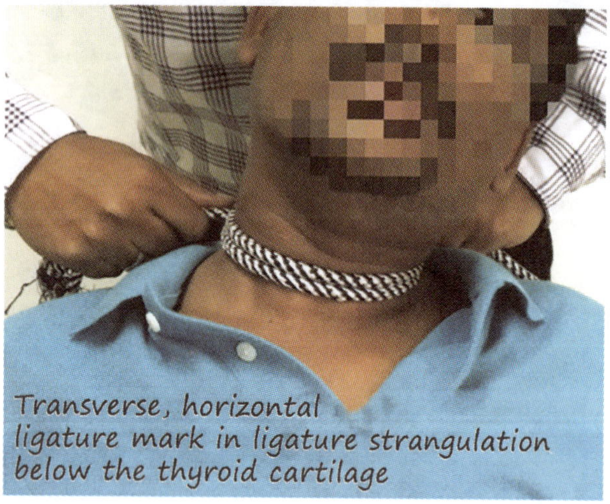

Transverse, horizontal ligature mark in ligature strangulation below the thyroid cartilage

Ligature strangulation—ligature mark

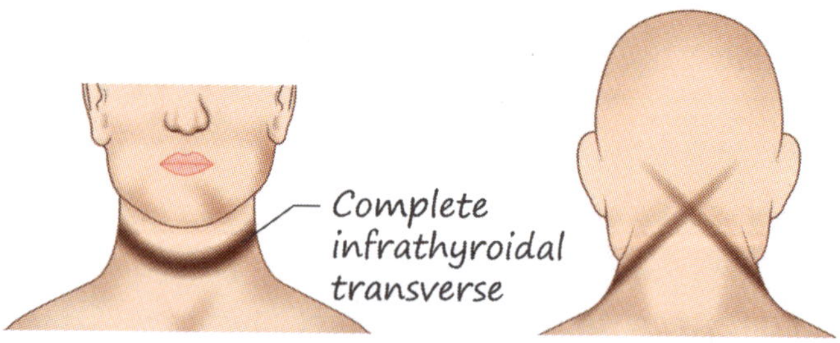

Neck Findings

Signs of asphyxia are more marked.

Ligature Mark

- Ligature mark is **transverse, completely encircling the neck, below the thyroid cartilage**^Q (usually).

- Base is reddish with ecchymosis.
- Fracture of the thyroid cartilage is more common[Q].
- Involuntary discharge of feces and urine is more common.

THROTTLING/MANUAL STRANGULATION (HANDS USED TO COMPRESS THE NECK)

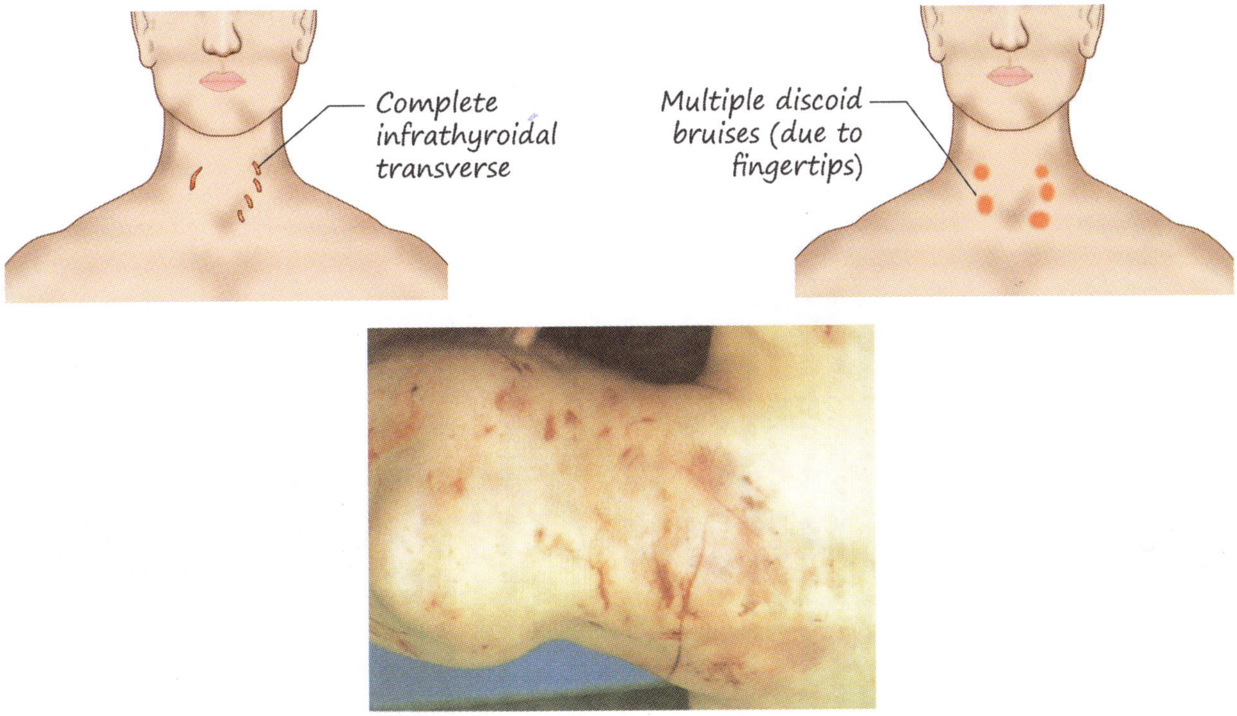

Signs of asphyxia are more evident.

Face congestion, petechial hemorrhages over the face, eyelids and temple present.

Neck Findings

- Externally, crescentic or linear finger nail abrasions[Q] are seen.
- **Multiple discoid bruises**[Q], due to compression by fingertips are seen.
- **Intense extravasation of blood in subcutaneous tissues under the external abrasions and bruises is the most significant internal sign**[Q].
- Adduction fracture[Q] of hyoid bone present.
- Thyroid cartilage superior horn fracture may be present.

> **Throttling**
> - **Homicidal throttling**[Q] **(always) > > Accidental throttling** (very rare)
> - **Suicidal throttling impossible**

BANSDOLA

- Constriction of the neck by **bamboo sticks**[Q], one across the back of the neck and another across the front.
- Both ends are tied with a rope due to which the victim is squeezed to death.

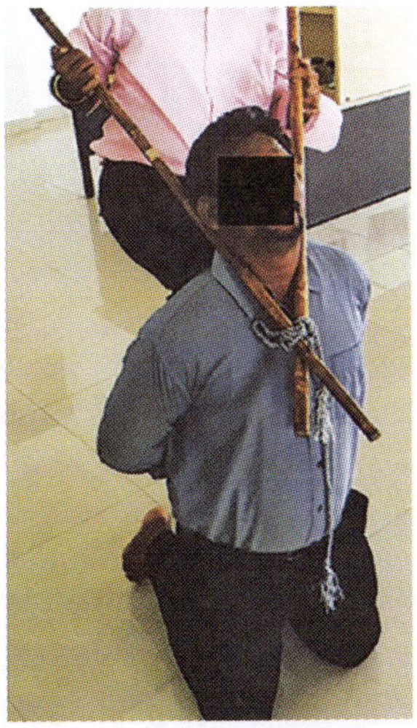

MUGGING

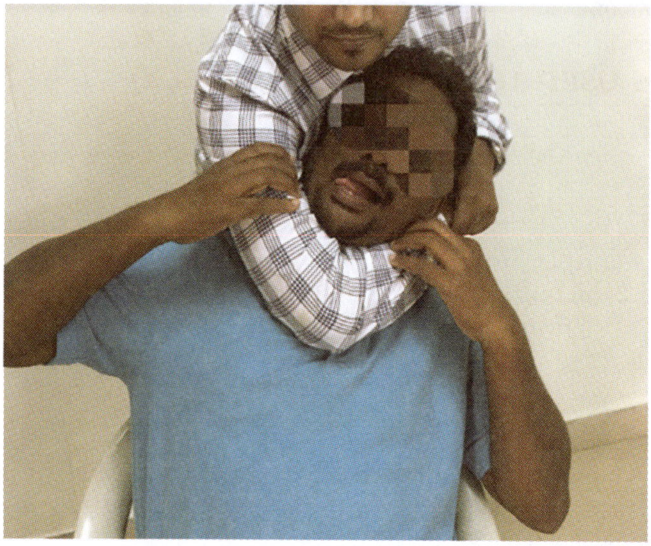

Strangulation of the neck by bending the elbow[Q] or forearm of the assailant.

GARROTING

- It is a form of strangulation[Q] of the neck by a thin ligature cord.
- The victim is attacked from behind without warning.
- A ligature is thrown over the neck and quickly tightened, by twisting it with a lever (rod, stick, ruler, etc.), which results in sudden loss of consciousness and collapse[Q].

Spanish method[Q] (type of garrotting)

- It was a method of judicial execution[Q] in Spain.
- Spanish windlass[Q]: A device used for garroting.
- It consists of an iron collar placed around the neck and tightened by a screw for strangulation.

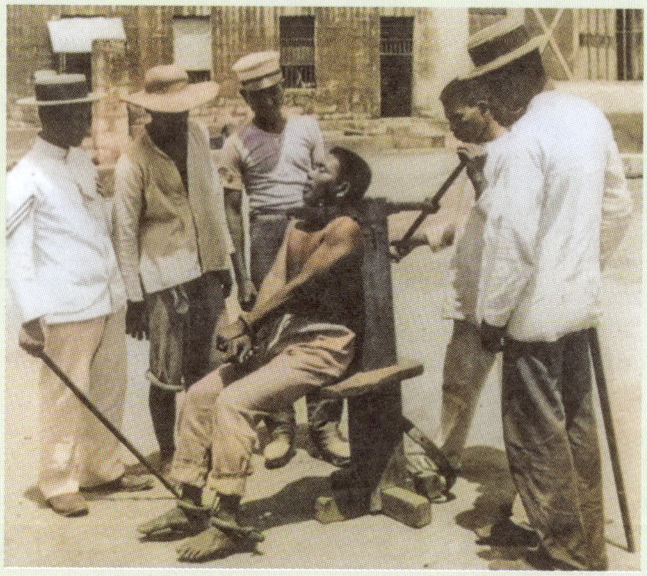

SUFFOCATION DEATHS

Smothering

- Asphyxia due to closure *of external air passages*[Q] (nose and mouth) by hand, cloth, etc.
- **Accidental/homicidal.**

Homicidal smothering	Accidental smothering
Mouth and nose closed by hands or clothes or pillow. **Postmortem findings:** • If smothered by hands, fingernail abrasions and bruises around the mouth and nostrils can be seen. • Injuries on the inside of the lips seen (contusions and laceration)	• Children may get smotheredwhile playing with plastic bags • Person may fall and be buried into finely divided materials like sand or grains.

Choking

- Asphyxia due to occlusion of internal air passages[Q] by a foreign object like coin, seeds, fish, etc.

Cause of death

Asphyxia[Q]

Vagal inhibition[Q]

Laryngeal spasm

- **Choking is usually accidental[Q]**

First aid: Heimlich's maneuver.

Café-Coronary (this term is a misnomer)

- Victim, who was apparently healthy, collapses suddenly dying while eating. Occurs during intoxication or drug influence.
- It mimics a heart attack and is usually seen in an intoxicated restaurant patron.
- A case of accidental choking[Q] wherein, a bolus of food produces complete obstruction of the larynx.
- **Cause of death:** Reflex cardiac arrest from 'vagal inhibition' as a consequence of stimulation of laryngeal nerve endings.

Gagging

- **Asphyxia due** to gag (rolled up cloth or paper balls) pushed into mouth and obstructing the pharynx.
- Almost always homicidal[Q]
- Victim is usually an infant or an elderly person.
- Even if the cloth is small, it may absorb saliva and swell, blocking the air entry.

Traumatic asphyxia/perthes syndrome

- Asphyxia due to mechanical fixation of chest[Q], so that the normal movements of chest wall are prevented[Q].

Causes

- Due to the collapse of the wall/house.
- Stampede by the crowd, running in panic
- Run over by a vehicle.

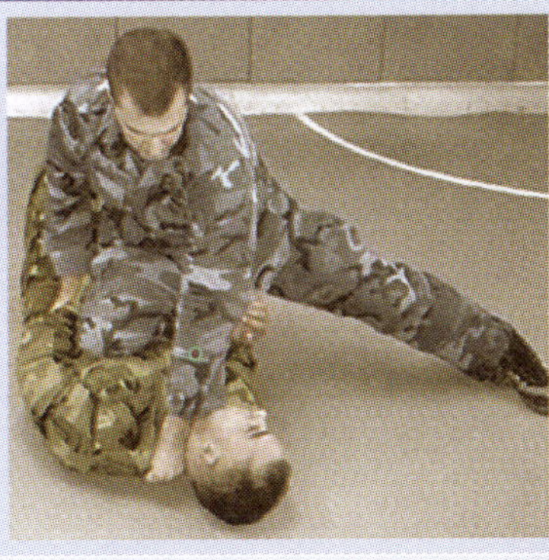

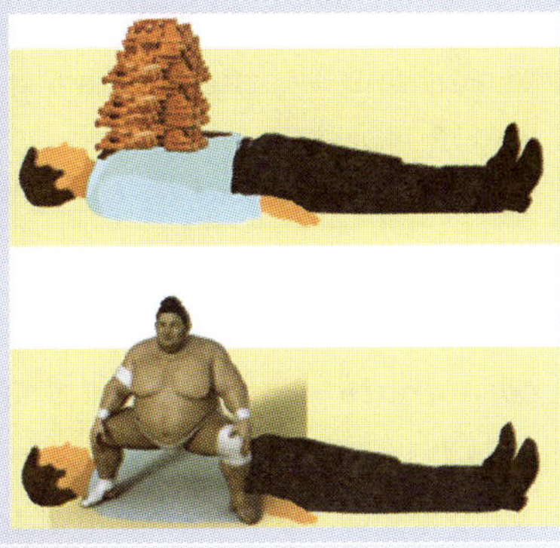

Postmortem examination

- **Masque ecchymotique[Q]**
  - Florid red or blue congestion of face and neck.
  - Demarcation line: Level of compression is indicated by a well-defined demarcating line between the discolored upper portion of body and the lower normal part.
- **Mostly accidental in nature.**

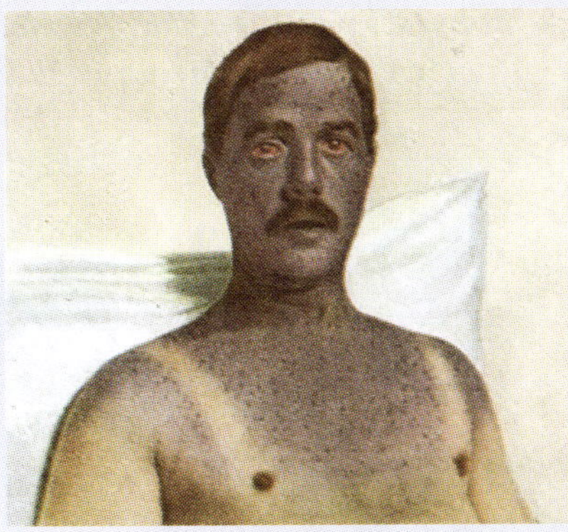

Positional/postural asphyxia: Positional asphyxia is due to abnormal body position that prevents adequate respiration/gas exchange.

Examples: Death in inverted crucifixion, Jack knife's position

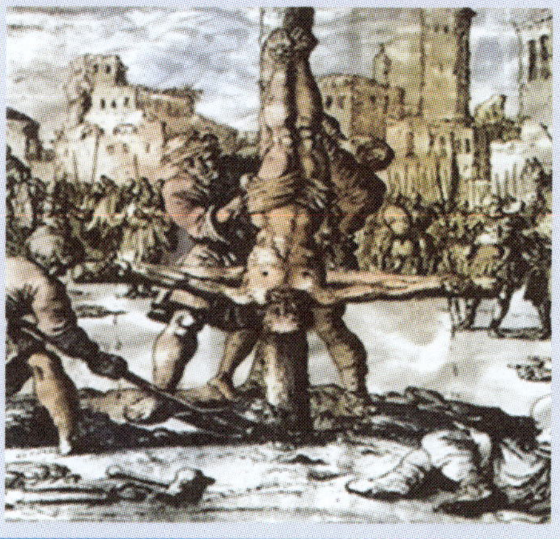

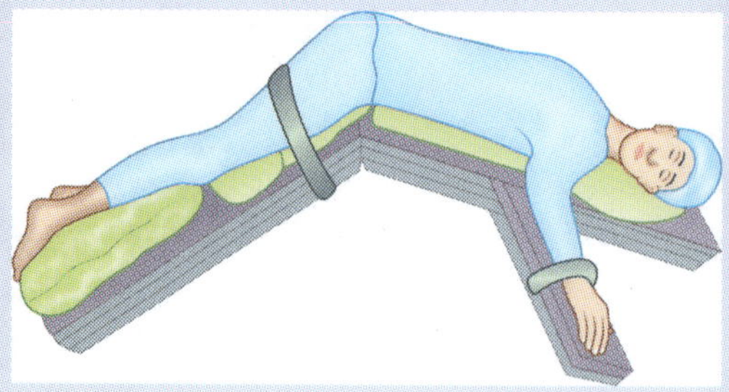

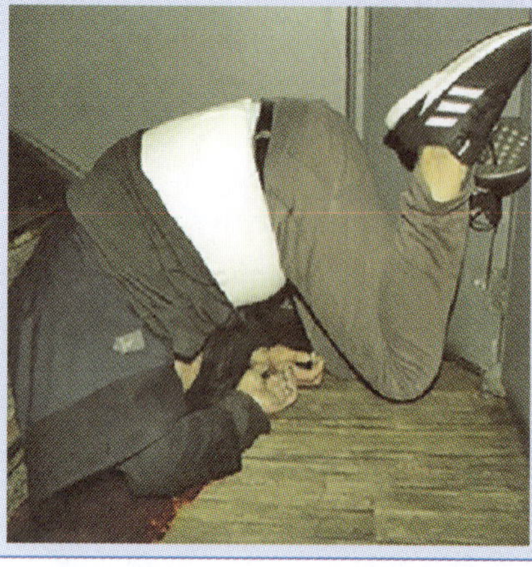

Overlaying

- Overlaying results from compression of the chest, nose and mouth to prevent breathing.
- A nursing mother, sharing a bed with her child, may roll over during sleep and occlude the air passages.
- **Purely accidental in nature.**

Burking

A combination of **homicidal smothering and traumatic asphyxia**[Q].

Method:

- Victims were invited, made to drink alcohol and thrown on the ground.
- William Burke would kneel or sit on the chest and close the nose and mouth with his hands, and William Hare used to pull him around the room by the feet till he is dead.

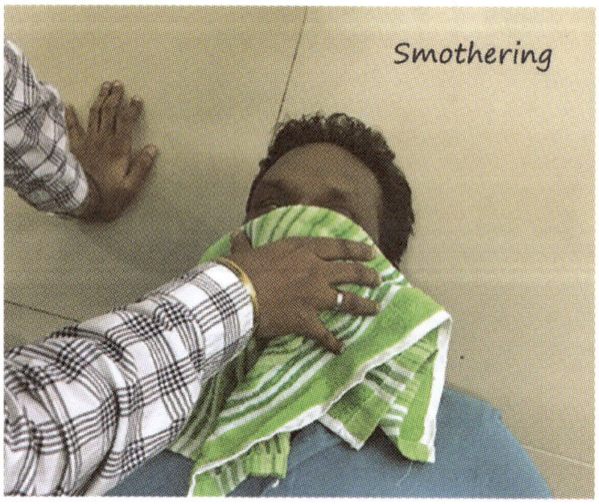

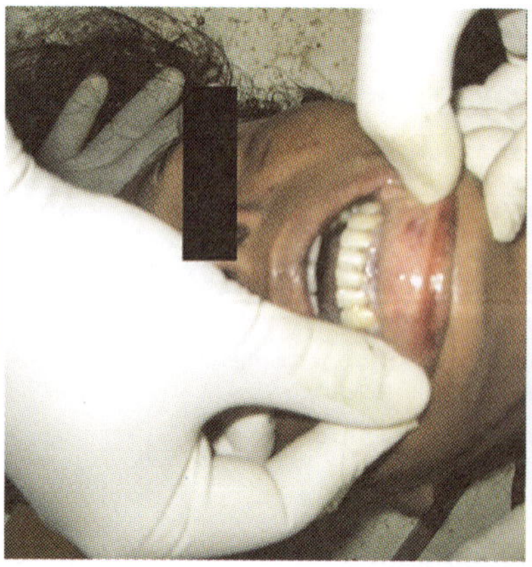

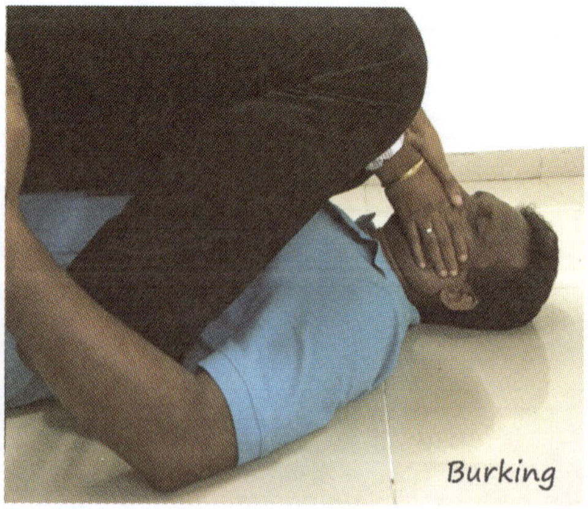

Bruises over the inner surface of the lips.

DROWNING

WHO Definition

Drowning is a process of respiratory impairment due to the submersion or immersion in liquid.

Types of Drowning

Typical drowning (primarily fluid entry into alveoli)	Atypical drowning (no fluid entry into alveoli)
Wet drowning	Dry drowning
Secondary drowning (near drowning syndrome)	Hydrocution

Atypical		Wet drowning
Hydrocution	**Dry drowning**	**Pathophysiology depends upon the amount of water aspirated**
Fall in cold water ↓ Nerve ending stimulation ↓ Vagal inhibition ↓ Cardiac arrest	Fall in water ↓ Sudden rush on water into pharynx ↓ Laryngeal spasm ↓ Asphyxia and death	(3–4 mL/KgBW) (MC) – Enters alveoli and washes away surfactants – Alveolar Collapse – Mismatch VP ratio – Cerebral Hypoxemia – Diffuse end organ damage/death

Wet Drowning 11 mL/kg (Pathophysiology depends upon the type of water)	
Fresh water (hypotonic)	Salt water (hypertonic)
Freshwater drowning	**Seawater drowning**

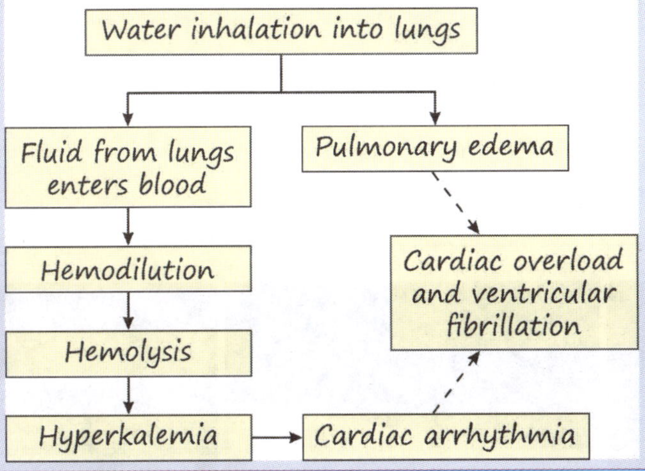

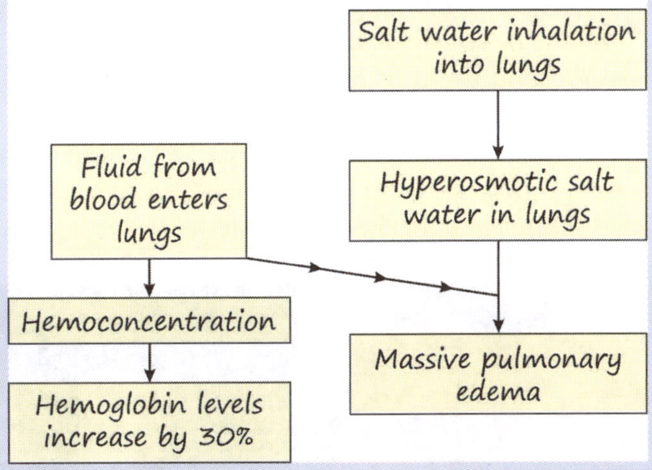

Note: Electrolyte imbalance is noted when amount of water aspirated is about 22 mL/kg

Hydrocution[Q]/Immersion Syndrome/Submersion Inhibition

- Occurs in drowning in cold water, which stimulates the vagal nerve endings[Q] at surface of the body or water striking the epigastrium or cold water entering the ear passage.
- Death results from sudden cardiac arrest[Q] due to **vagal inhibition of heart**[Q].

Postmortem Appearance

Livor mortis:
- In stagnant water: Face, upper part of the chest, lower arms and feet[Q]
- In moving water: No appearance

Froth in drowning (A sign of antemortem drowning)
- A fine, white, lathery froth[Q] is seen at the mouth and nostrils.
- Balloon/mushroom-like mass from the mouth and nostrils.
- If wiped away, it gradually reappears, on applying pressure on the chest.

Cadaveric spasm (surest sign of antemortem drowning[Q])

Grass, gravel, sand, weeds or aquatic vegetation held firmly in clenched hands due to cadaveric spasm[Q].

Cutis anserina (Goose skin/goose bumps/horripilation)
- Due to contraction of erector pilorum muscles.
- **Nonspecific[Q] for drowning.** (Can also occur in rigor mortis of erector muscles).

Washerwomen's hand (nonspecific sign)
- Wrinkled, sodden, bleached appearance of skin.
- **Site:** Palms, palmar aspect of fingers and soles of feet including plantar surface of toes.
- Due to imbibition of water into its outer layers.
- **Time:** First seen in the fingertips by 3–4 hours and whole hand by 24 hours.

! ATTENTION: Froth formation will not be seen in case of dry drowning and hydrocution.

Internal findings

- **Lungs:**
  - Voluminous, distended and show ballooning.
  - Distended lungs show rib markings.
- **Emphysema aquosum**[Q]
  - Intra-alveolar edema with thinning of intra-alveolar septa and bullae noted.
  - Copious frothy fluid exudes
  - Presence of sand particles in the airway[Q]
- **Paltauf's hemorrhage**
  - Mottled areas of hemorrhage in lungs.
  - Rupture of alveoli due to forced expiration.
  - Mostly seen in the **lower lobes**[Q] on anterior surface and margins of lungs.
  - Presence of water in stomach and small intestine
  - Temporal bone hemorrhages

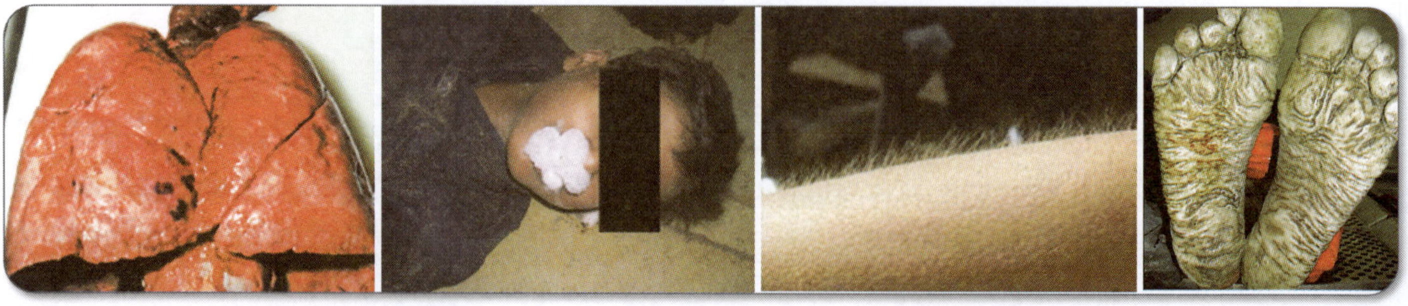

Airway

- Presence of sand, mud, aquatic vegetations in the trachea and lower bronchial tree are characteristic **positive findings of antemortem drowning**[Q].
- Water in the small intestine—This is regarded as **positive evidence of death by drowning** as it depends on peristaltic movement which is antemortem.

Middle ear (Ueno's sign)

- Presence of water and hemorrhage in middle ear is one of the positive proofs of antemortem drowning.

Emphysema aquosum[Q]
- Lungs contains both water and froth
- Occurs when the conscious victim[Q] of drowning struggles for survival

Edema aquosum[Q]
- Mere flooding of lungs with the airless water and no formation of froth
- Occurs when the person is unconscious[Q] at the time of drowning

Hydrostatic lung[Q]
- Passive filling of lungs with water due to hydrostatic pressure
- Occurs when dead body is thrown into water

Laboratory Investigations

Diatom Test

- Diatoms are microscopic unicellular algae, which secrete silica[Q] skeletons called frustules.
- They are chemically inert and almost indestructible, being resistant to strong acids.
- Diatoms of size 60μ enters the circulation.

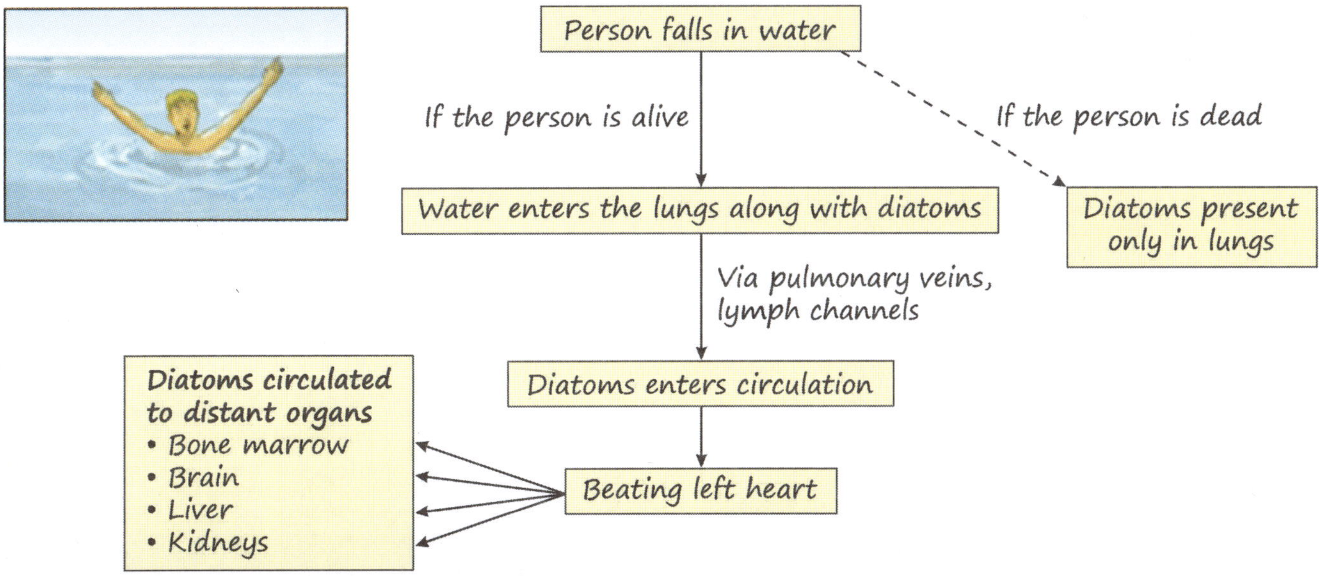

- Presence of diatoms in the distant tissues like **bone marrow of femur**[Q] (best site for analysis) is the proof of **antemortem drowning**
- The test is negative in dead bodies thrown in the water and in dry drowning[Q].

Gettler Test

Based on chloride content[Q] **of blood in heart chambers**.

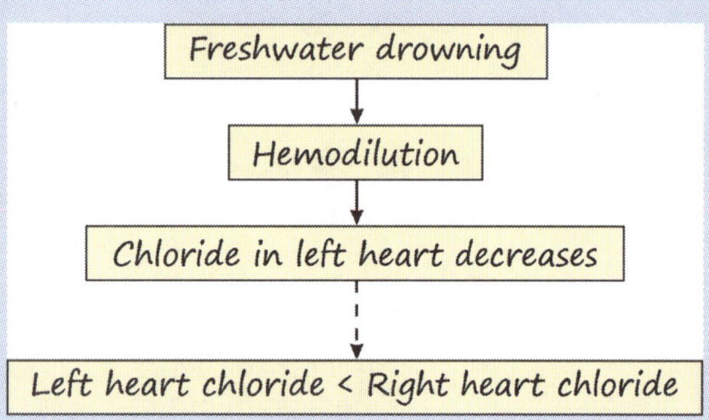

Normally, the chloride content of the right and left side of heart is nearly same, about 600 mg/100 mL.

- If the difference is 25 mg% or more, it is suggestive of antemortem drowning.
- In freshwater drowning, chloride reduces by 50% in left ventricle.
- In seawater drowning, chloride increases by 30–40% in left ventricle.

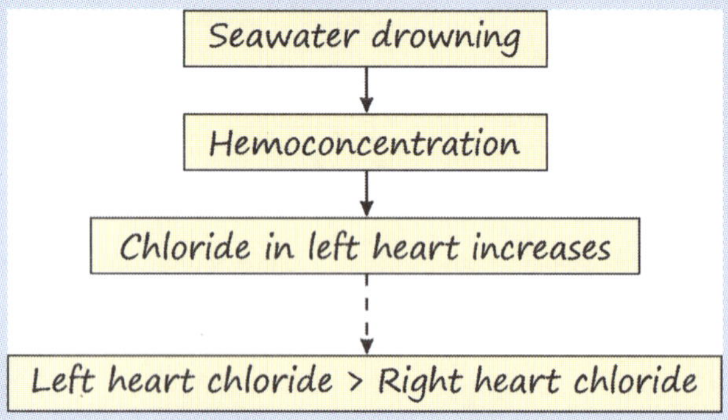

No change in chloride content of heart:

- Drowning due to laryngeal spasm or vagal inhibition.
- Putrefaction.
- Patent foramen ovale.

4. FORENSIC TRAUMATOLOGY

MECHANICAL INJURIES

Blunt force injuries (ground, stone, hammer)	Sharp force: Light cutting weapon (surgical blade)	Sharp force: Heavy cutting weapon (chopper, axe)	Sharp force: Pointed weapon (kitchen knife, screw driver, pencil)
Abrasion (scratch) Contusion (bruise) Laceration[Q] (skin tear) Fracture of bones	Incised[Q] (cut injury)	Chop injury	Stab injury[Q]

ABRASION

- Destruction of superficial layers of the skin (partial epidermis) only.
- No/**slight bleeding**[Q], heal rapidly and **no scar formation**[Q].

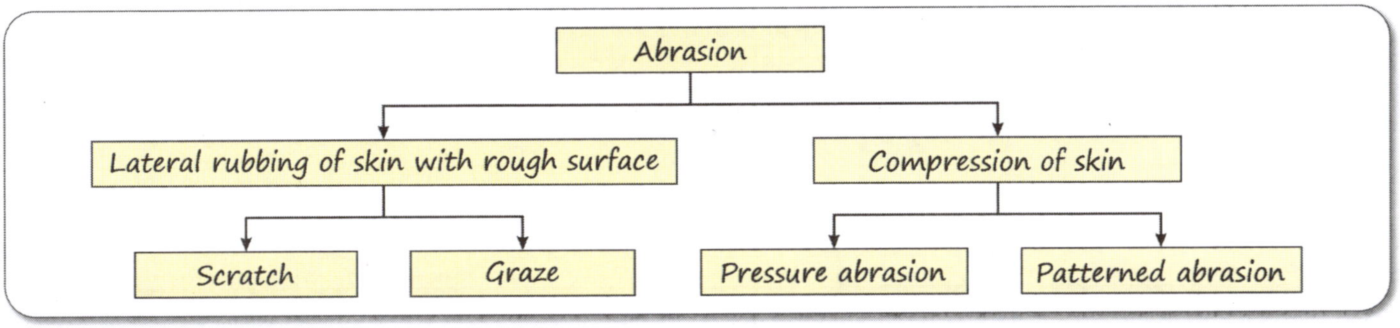

Scratch
- **Linear abrasion** caused by pointed or sharp object
- **Finger nail**[Q]/thorn/pin

Graze
- **Most common** type[Q] of abrasion
- Friction with rough surface over **wider area**
- **In road traffic accidents**[Q]
- Multiple uneven, **longitudinal parallel lines**[Q]
- Also called **brush burn/sliding abrasion/grinding abrasion**

Pressure
- **Pressure over the skin with crushing of epithelium**
- **Ligature mark**[Q] in hanging and strangulation

Patterned
- **Crushing of epithelium and Pattern of the weapon is imprinted** on the skin
- Ligature mark
- Teeth bite marks
- **Tread marks of tyre**[Q]

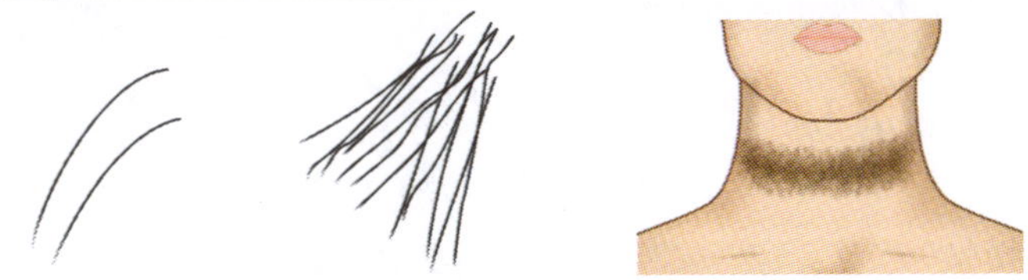

Linear scratch — Graze abrasion uneven longitudinal lines over wider area — Pressure abrasion

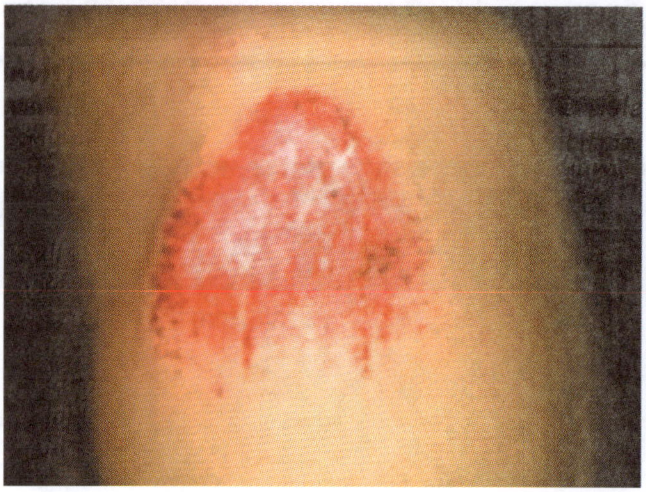

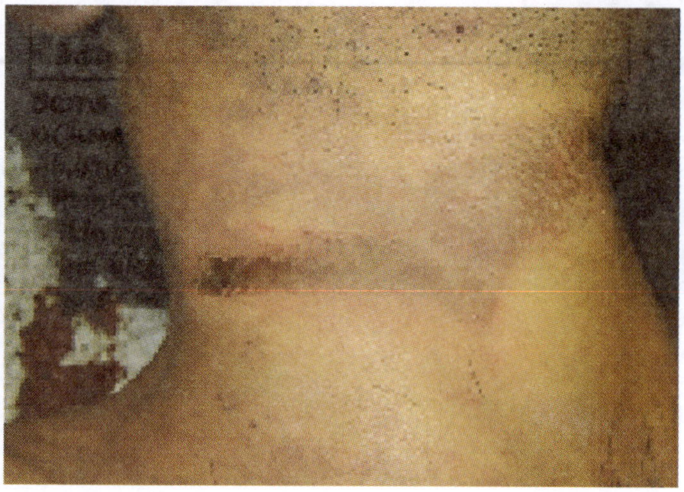

Direction of force

Heaping of epithelium or epithelial tag: Surface epithelium is scrapped and deposited at the tail end of the abrasion[Q]

Time since injury from abrasion

Mnemonic: RRRBBB—R^3B^3

R – Raw without scab (fresh)	–	<12 hours
R – Reddish scab[Q]	–	>12 hours
R B – Reddish brown scab[Q]	–	2–3 days
B – Brown scab	–	4–5 days
B – Black scab	–	6–7 days

- Abrasion heals from the periphery by growth of new epithelial cells
- After 7 days, scab falls off, leaving depigmented area underneath
- Usually abrasions are simple hurt (as they are superficial) except corneal abrasion, which may cause visual restriction (grievous hurt)

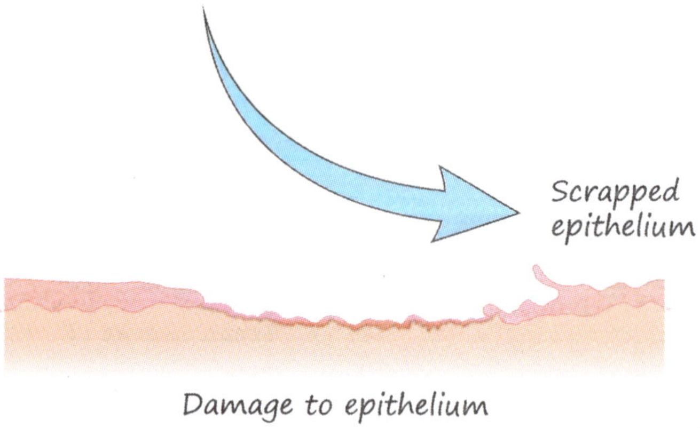

Medicolegal Significance of Abrasions (Medicolegally Most Significant Wound)

- Abrasions give an idea about the **direction of force**[Q].
- Patterned abrasions are helpful to find out the causative weapon.
- **Age of injury**[Q] can be determined.
- In open wounds, dirt or sand is usually present which is used to connect to the scene of crime.
- Manner of Injury: smothering (perioral abrasion); throttling (fingernail abrasions in neck).

Antemortem versus Postmortem Abrasions

Features	Antemortem abrasions	Postmortem abrasions
Site	**Anywhere on the body**	Bony prominences
Scab formation	Present	Absent
Color changes	Present[Q]	Absent, mostly yellowish without any change
Vital reaction	Present[Q]	Absent

CONTUSION/BRUISE

Contusion is the extravasation of blood[Q] under the skin due to rupture of blood vessels, usually capillaries, as a result of blunt force injury.

Contusion is present not only in the skin, but also in internal organs—lung, brain or muscle.

Blunt trauma to skin
↓
Dermal vessels rupture
↓
Bleeding in surrounding tissue
Extravasation
↓
Swelling and discoloration of skin
Contusion

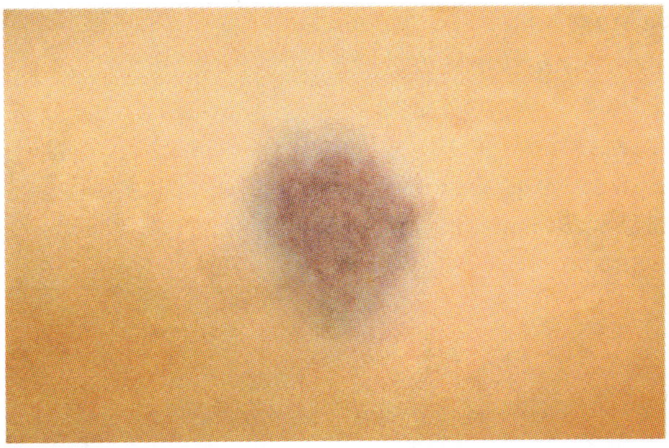

Types of Contusion

Type	Description
Superficial/intradermal bruise	Readily Visible soon after the impact
Deep bruise Delayed bruise or come out bruise	**Location:** Below deep fascia. May present out after a few hours/days.

Ectopic bruise/Percolated bruise/migratory bruise

- At a **site other than the site of injury**, e.g., black eyes.
- Thus, site of bruise does not always indicate the site of injury.

Black eye/spectacle hematoma[Q]

Bruising around the eye

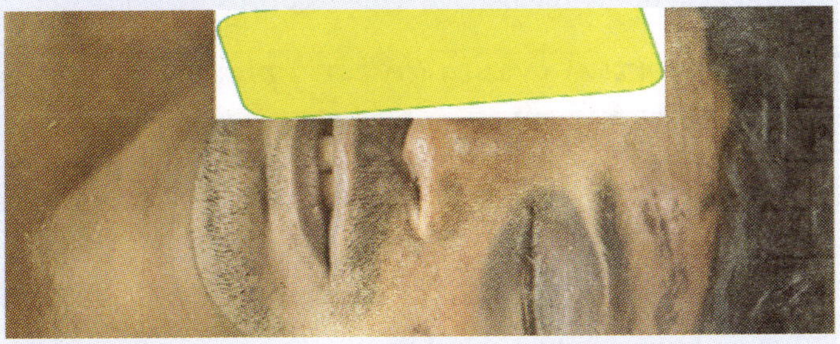

Battle's sign

- Bruising over the mastoid process (mastoid ecchymosis).
- Seen in 12-24 hours of injury.
- Indicates fracture of middle cranial fossa.

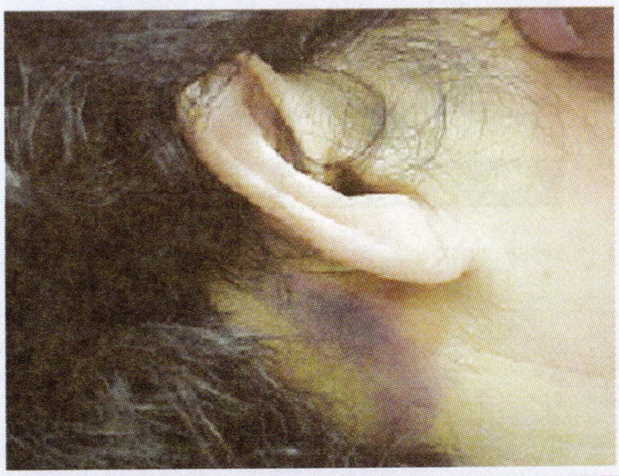

Contd...

Patterned bruise[Q]: Patterned bruise indicates the nature of the weapon

Railway line or tramline type[Q]	Doughnut bruise	Six penny bruise	Butterfly bruise
• Blows with a **rod, stick** or a whip produce **two parallel, linear hemorrhage.** • The intervening skin appears pale. • The diameter of the pale area may indicate the diameter of the weapon.	Caused by spherical object.	• Bruise looks like a six penny coin. • Caused by finger tip pressure on skin. • Seen in manual strangulation and child abuse	• Caused by skin pinching. • In children, indicates child abuse.

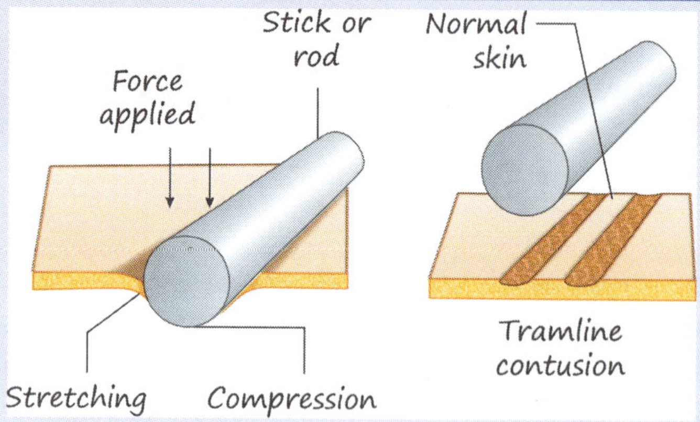

Aging or Dating of Bruise

1. Color of bruise. 2. Spectrometry. 3. Histology. 4. Pearl stain reaction.

- As bruises heal, there is a gradual destruction and removal of the extravasated blood.
- Color change starts at the periphery and extends inwards to the center.

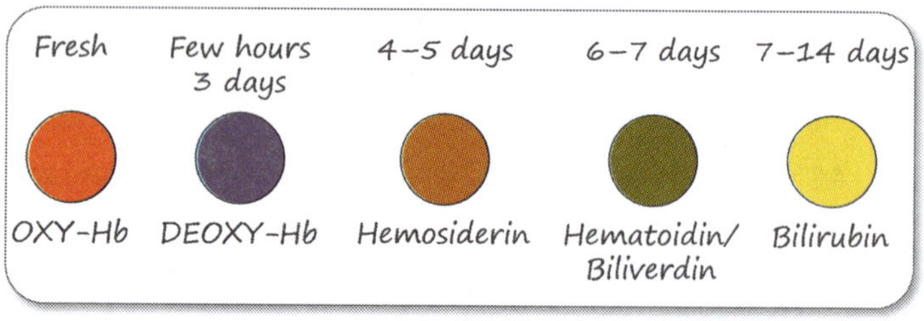

Oxyhemoglobin (red)
↓
Deoxyhemoglobin (blue)
↓
Hemosiderin (brown/violet)
↓
Hematoidin/biliverdin (green)
↓
Bilirubin (yellow)

Extra Edge

- Sites where **NO** color changes seen—subconjunctival hemorrhage (due to continuous exposure of air)
- Multiple bruises of different ages in a same person is a feature of child abuse[Q].

Differential Diagnosis of Contusion

- Postmortem lividity (in early phases)

Character	PM lividity	Contusion
Site	**Dependent parts**	**Anywhere**
Margins	**Well defined**	**Ill defined**
Extravasation	**Absent**	**Present**
Blanching	**Present**	**Absent**
Color changes	**Absent**	**Present**
On incision, pour water	**Washes away**	**Remains**

- **Artificial bruise/Pseudo bruise**
  - Certain irritant substances and plant juices are applied on the skin to mimic artificial bruise.

Difference between True Bruise and Pseudo/False Bruise

Character	True bruise	Pseudo bruise
Cause	Blunt Trauma	**Plant poisons like** **S** – **Semicarpus** **P** – **Plumbago** **M** – (Madar) Calotropis Mnemonic: **Social Preventive Medicine**
Location	Anywhere on the body[Q]	**Accessible parts** of body Like forearm, thighs, abdomen
Blister/vesication	Not present	Present[Q]
Itching	Not Present	Present[Q]
Color changes	Characteristic of true bruise (**color changes** as it heals)	Absent
Contents	Blood	Acrid serum[Q]
Chemical analysis	Negative	Chemical/plant juice detected

LACERATION

- Tissues are torn as a result of application of blunt force.
- Tissues may be skin, mucous membrane, muscles or internal organs.
- Laceration is three-dimensional (length, breadth and depth)

General Features of Laceration

- Irregular shape[Q]
- Irregular[Q] and uneven margins, torn edges
- Contused edges[Q]
- **Floor of laceration shows the following features**
    - **Tissue bridges** (tissue, blood vessels and nerves bridging across the gap of the wound)
    - **Crushed**[Q]
    - **Less hemorrhage**[Q] because of crushed blood vessels.
    - Foreign particles like mud may be seen embedded in the wound, which gives clue about the scene of crime

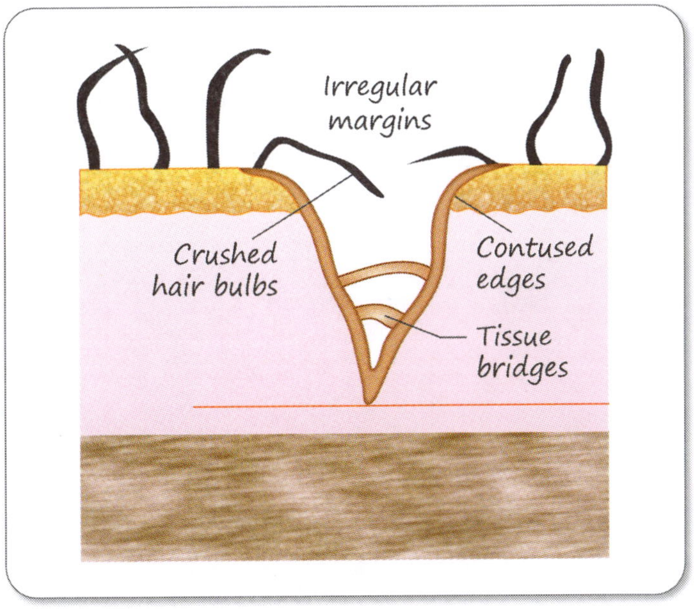

Types of Laceration

Split	stretch	Tear	Avulsion/Grinding	CUT laceration
• Skin **crushed between two hard surfaces,** i.e. the weapon and the underlying bone • Incised like/ Incised looking laceration[Q] Naked eye: margins may appear regular On magnifying lens: Crushed floor and irregular edges. **Laceration looking an incision = Incised looking laceration** **Common sites:** Bony prominences, i.e., scalp, face, forehead, cheeks, chin, iliac crest, shin bone	• Heavy blunt force at an angle to the skin ↓ Pressure with pull force ↓ **Overstretching of the skin** till it ruptures • Striae-like lacerations or stretch mark-like lacerations	• Tearing of skin and SC tissue due to localized impact	Grinding compression force/tangential force/ shearing force • Seen in **Run over**[Q] injuries • **Direction of force**[Q] can be determined The severity of avulsion ranges from skin flaps (minor) to degloving (moderate) and amputation of a finger or limb (severe). • **Flaying**[Q]: The rotating force of a wheel tears off the skin over a large area—flaying, and most frequently on the legs. • **Degloving injury:** A severe type where a large area of skin and subcutaneous tissue is rolled off a limb (like a glove). • **Scalping:** A large area of skin and SC tissue is rolled off the scalp (especially when the hair is trapped in machinery).	Caused by heavy cutting with blunt edges like axe.

Medicolegal Importance

- Usually accidental or homicidal.
- Foreign particles in lacerations help in identifying the weapon or crime scene.
- Direction of force (avulsion laceration).

INCISED WOUND: (CUT/SLASH/SLICE)

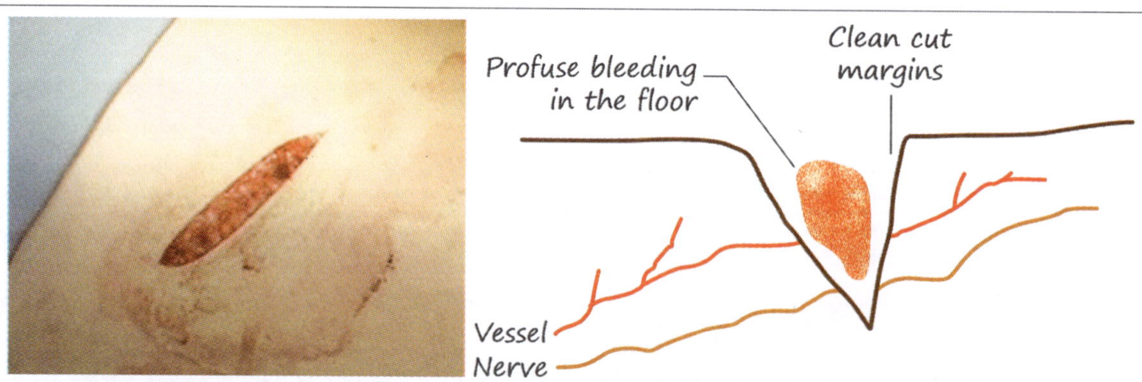

Character

- **Margins:** Clean cut[Q], regular[Q]
- **Floor: Cut vessels and hair bulb**
- **Profuse hemorrhage**[Q] due to cut vessels

Dimensions

- **Length:** It is the maximum dimension[Q]
- **Depth/direction:**
  - **Head end:** Deeper at the beginning of the wound
  - **Tail end:** Shallow at the termination[Q]

Tailing[Q]

- Tailing it is a feature of **incised wound**
- Usually deeper at the beginning (head end) and toward termination, the cut becomes progressively shallow, known as tailing of the wound.
- **Direction of force**[Q] can be determined.

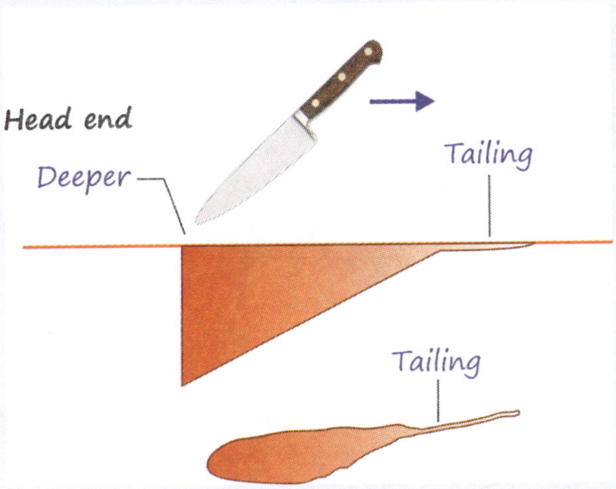

Beveling cuts

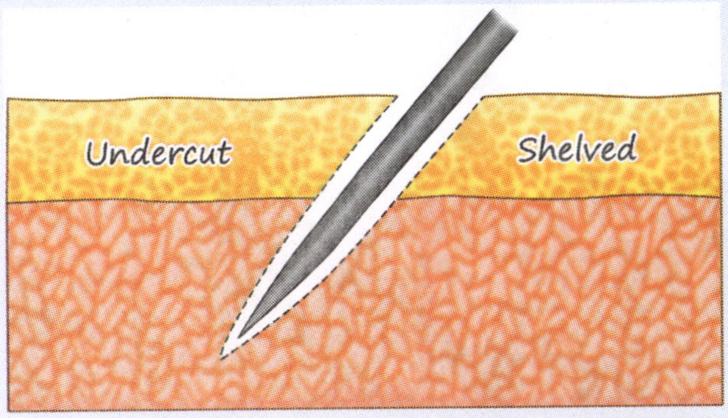

- Produced by oblique cuts[Q]
- If the blade enters obliquely, tissues will be visible at one margin and other margin will be undermined.
- Indicates **homicidal nature.**
- **Direction** of application of the weapon, and **the relative position of assailant and the victim** can also be determined.

Hesitation Cuts/Tentative Cuts/Feeler's Strokes/Intentional Cuts

- Indicates suicidal nature[Q] of the wound.
- Multiple, small, superficial, parallel cuts noticed over the accessible body parts[Q].
- Sites: Over throat, wrist, elbow, front of chest and abdomen.

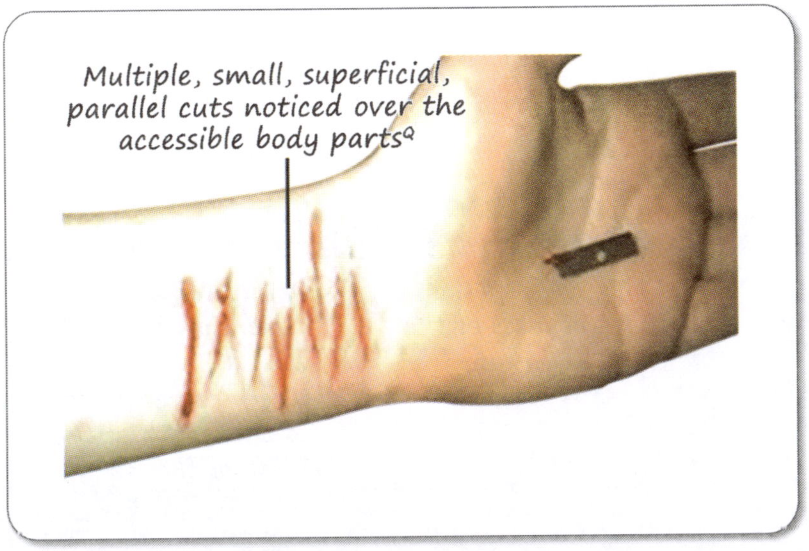

Medicolegal importance

- Nature of force: Sharp.
- Manner of injury: **Suicidal (hesitation cuts), accidental or homicidal (beveled cuts/cuts on face, genitals etc).**
- Age of the injury from healing.
- Direction of force **(tailing)**

Incised wound

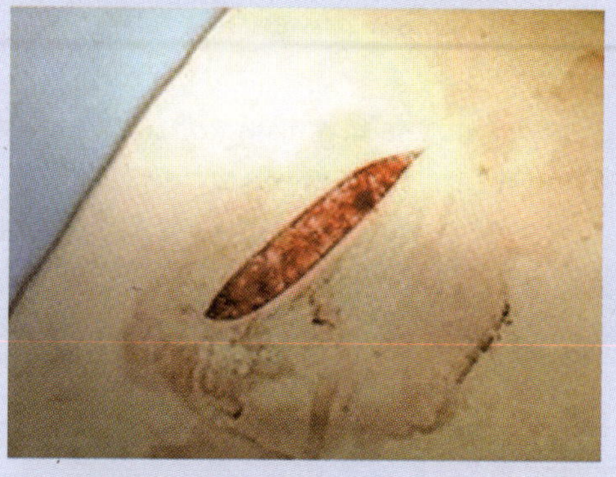

Laceration

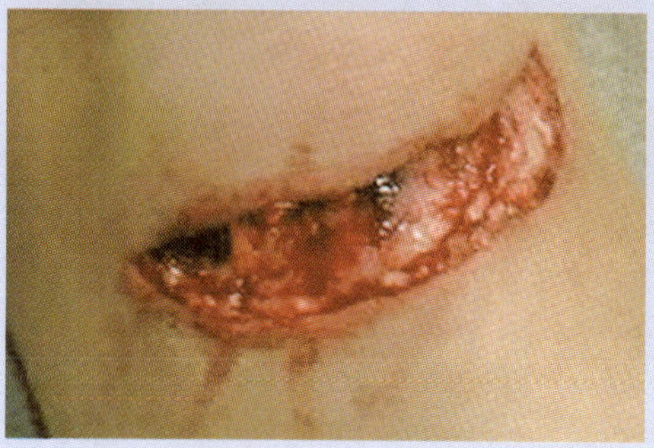

Characters	Laceration	Incised wound
Margins	Irregular, edges contused	Clean cut, regular
Tissue bridges	Present	Absent
Tailing	Absent	Present
Bleeding	Less (due to crushing of vessels)	More (due to cutting of vessels)

CHOP WOUND

- Caused by a blow with the sharp-cutting heavy weapon (hatchet, axe etc)
- **Deep gaping wounds**[Q].
- **Undermining** occurs in the direction toward which the chop is made.
- Underlying fracture present. +
- Most of the injuries are **homicidal**.

STAB WOUND (PUNCTURED WOUND)

- Produced from penetration of weapons with pointed ends.
- **Depth**[Q] **is the maximum dimension** of stab wound.

Characteristics

Margins	Length	Breadth	Depth
Edges of the wound are clean cut.	Length is slightly less than the width of the weapon because of stretching of the skin.	Roughly corresponds to the thickness of the blade.	• Depth is the **greatest dimension** of a stab wound. • Depth corresponds to the length of the blade of the weapon entering the body.

Types

- **Penetrating wound:** Weapon enters into the body cavity producing only one entry wound.
- **Perforating wound:** Weapon after entering into cavity and coming out through the other side, producing two wounds (entry wound and exit wound).

Features	Entry wounds	Exit wounds
Margins	Inverted[Q]	Everted[Q]
Size	Larger	Smaller

Shape of Stab Wound

Single edge knife			Double edged knife	Screw driver	Dining fork
Tear drop	Wedge/ triangle	Fish tailing	Oval/spindle Both angles are sharp		○○○○

Langer's Lines or Cleavage Lines

- Langer's lines are the imaginary lines representing the **pattern of collagen fiber**[Q] arrangements on the skin.
- Langer's lines determine the **Gaping**[Q] of stab injury.
- Wound perpendicular to the cleavage lines—gaping will be more.
- Wound parallel to the cleavage lines—gaping will be less.

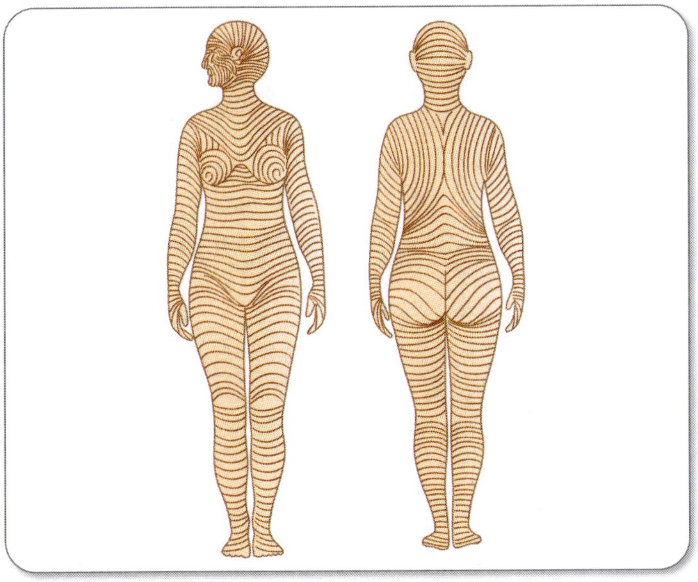

Active defense injuries	Passive defense injuries
Seen when the victim tries to grasp the weapon. Location: palms, the flexor sides of the fingers and more common in the web between the thumb and index finger.	Seen when the victim raises the hands or arms for protection. Location: Ulnar surfaces of forearms, wrists, knuckles and the back of the hands

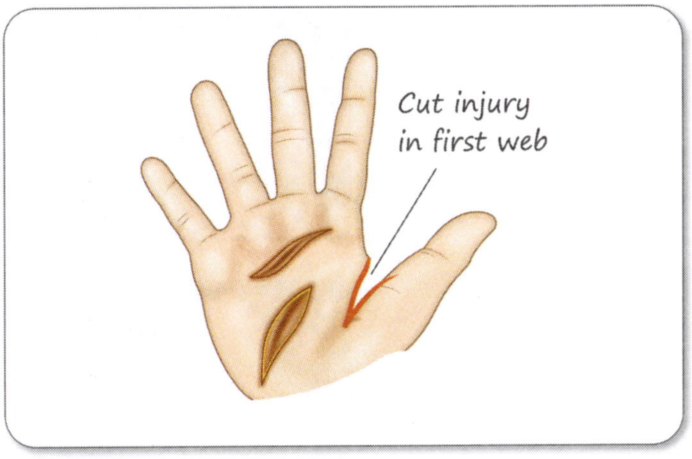

The presence of defense wounds indicate **homicidal nature**[Q] of the injuries, but not mandatory.

Defense/Protective Wounds

- Defense/protective wounds result from **victim's spontaneous instinctive reaction**[Q] toward self-protection.
- If the weapon is blunt, bruises and abrasions are produced.
- If the weapon is sharp, the injuries will depend upon the type of attack, whether stabbing or cutting.

Harakiri (Seppuku)

- Method of committing suicide by Japanese samurai warriors.
- Suicidal stab injury abdomen.
- A single large abdominal stab wound is inflicted by a short sword on the left side, drawing the blade across to the right side and then turning it upward producing an L-shaped cut.
- Death is due to sudden evisceration[Q] of the internal organs and circulatory collapse.

REGIONAL INJURIES

Types of Skull Fractures

Fractures of Skull Vault

Type of fracture	Causative force	Description
Fissure Fracture Blows with an agent having a relatively broad striking surface[Q]	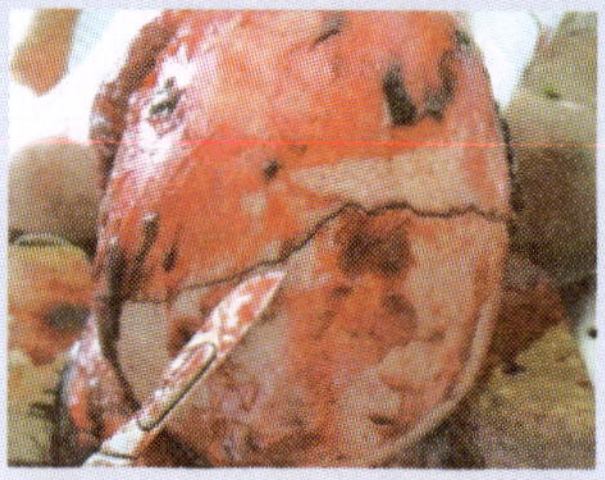	• **Most common fracture**[Q]. • **Thin linear cracks** without any displacement of the fragments. • Difficult to detect in X-ray, and can only be detected at autopsy.
Depressed fracture **Heavy weapon with a small striking surface**[Q] Like hammer	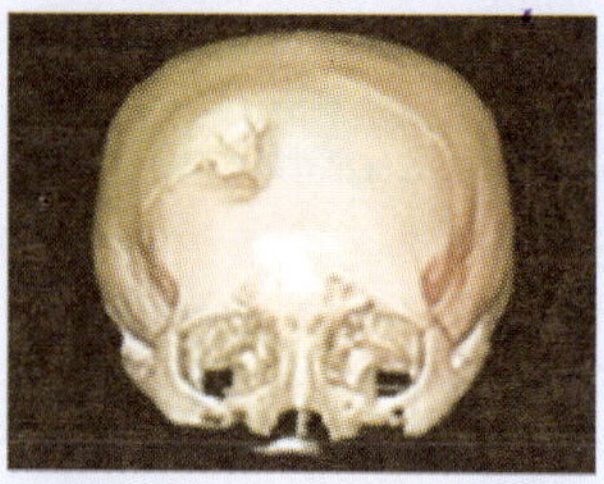	• Fractured bone is depressed inward into the cranial cavity. • The fractured segment resembles **the pattern of the striking surface of the weapon**[Q]. • It is also called **'fracture ala signature' (signature fracture)**.
Comminuted fracture	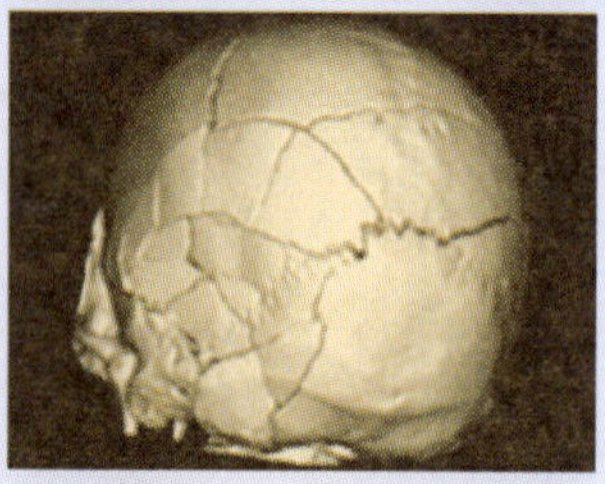	• Two or more fracture lines intersect and divide the bone into three or more fragments.[Q] • When there is no displacement of fragments, it resembles a spider's web or mosaic.
Pond fracture (indented fracture) **Obstetric forceps**[Q]	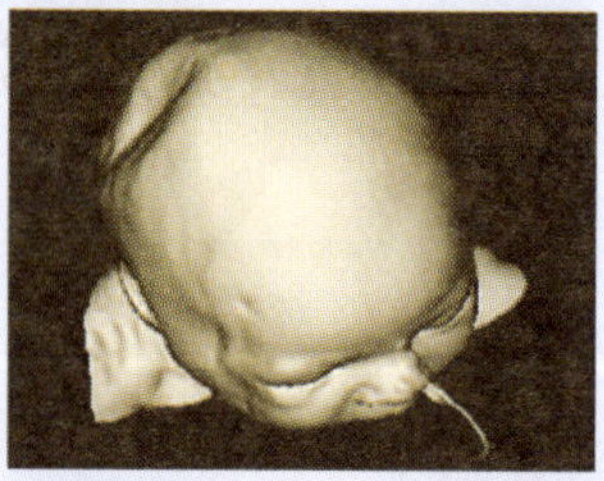	• A simple dent in the skull without a fracture line. • Dura and brain are not damaged. • Occurring **only in the skull of infants and children**[Q] due to pliability. • Also known as ping-pong fracture.
Diastatic/sutural fracture	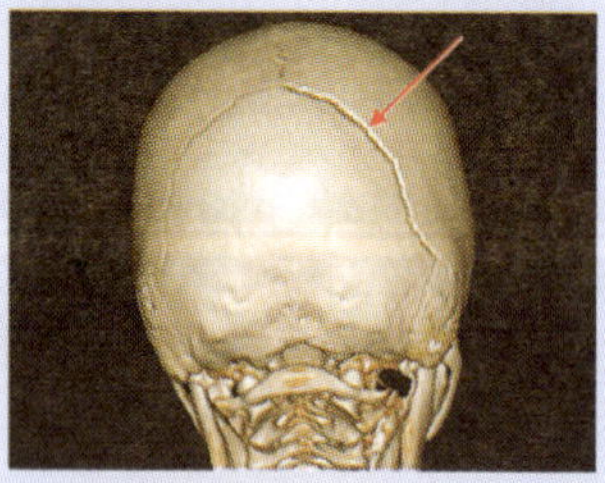	• Separation of skull sutures[Q]. • Common in sagittal suture. • Occurring in the skull of children and young adults.
Gutter fracture **Oblique bullet wounds**[Q]	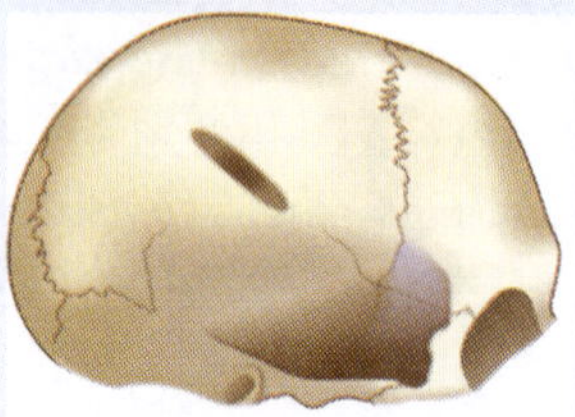	When a part of the thickness of the skull bone is removed so as to form a gutter/channel/trench.

Skull Base Fractures

Ring or foramen fracture • **Fall from a height**$_Q$ landing on feet or buttocks • Fall of heavy load on head Heavy blow to chin	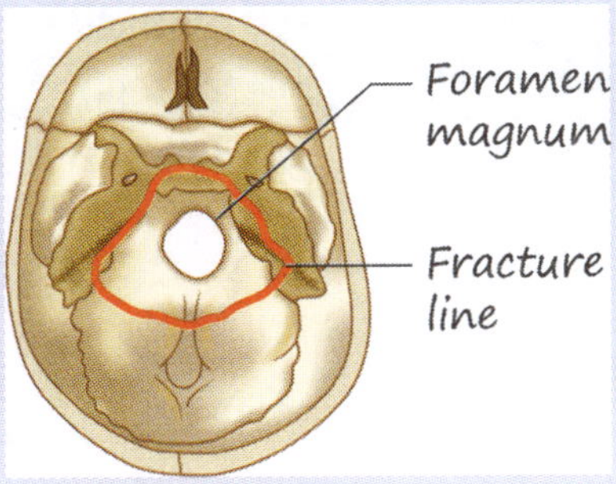	• It is a type of fissure fracture that encircles the base of **skull around the foramen magnum**[Q]. • As a result, the skull gets separated from the spine.
Hinge/transverse fracture With heavy blows or side impacts to head.	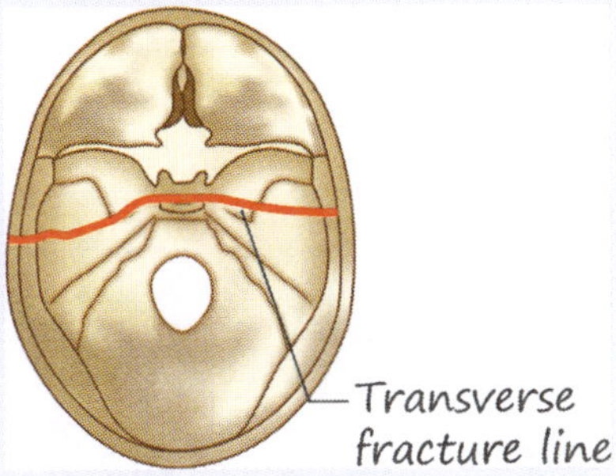	• Linear fracture separating the **skull into two halves, creating a hinge ('nodding face' sign)**[Q]. • The fracture line extends from petrous ridge on one side to the contralateral petrous ridge through sella turcica. • It is also called '**motorcyclists fracture**'. 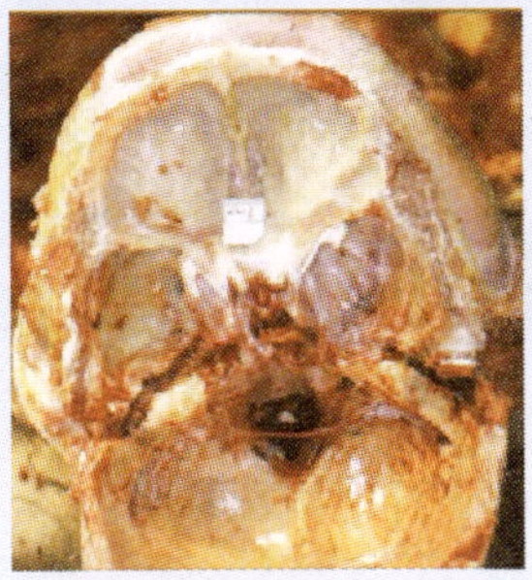

Coup and Contrecoup Injury

- ***Coup injury*** is one which occurs immediately beneath the area of impact.
- ***Contrecoup injury*** means that the brain injury opposite to the site of impact.
- Seen when head is free and mobile.
- It is caused when the moving head is suddenly decelerated by hitting a firm surface, e.g. striking of the head on the ground during a fall.
- When a person falls with his occiput hitting the ground, he may sustain injury at the occipital lobes (coup injury) and a more prominent injury to the frontal lobes (contrecoup injury).

Possibilities

Coup	Contrecoup
Mild/nil injury	Severe injury.
Occipital fall	Frontal lobe contusion (m/c).
Frontal impact	No occipital injury as inner surface of occipital bone is smooth.
Temporal lobe (one side)	• Opposite temporal lobe. • Contralateral surface of ipsilateral lobe (opposite surface of same lobe).

INTRACRANIAL HEMORRHAGES

	Extradural hemorrhage	Subdural hemorrhage	Subarachnoid hemorrhage	Intracerebral hemorrhage
Location	Between the skull and dura	Between dura and arachnoid	Between arachnoid and pia	Within the brain parenchyma
Most common vessel affected	**Middle meningeal artery**[Q]	**Bridging veins**[Q]	**Arterial aneurysms**[Q] **AV malformations**	Lenticulostriate branch of MCA

Extradural Hemorrhage

- Mostly traumatic in origin, and unilateral.
- Common in adults between 20 and 40 years.

Blow trauma to the side of head (pterion—temporoparietal region)
↓
Fracture of temporal bone (mostly fissure)
↓
Rupture of middle meningeal artery
↓
Bleeding in the extradural space
↓
Brain compression, increased ICT
↓
Brain stem involvement
↓
Death due to respiratory failure

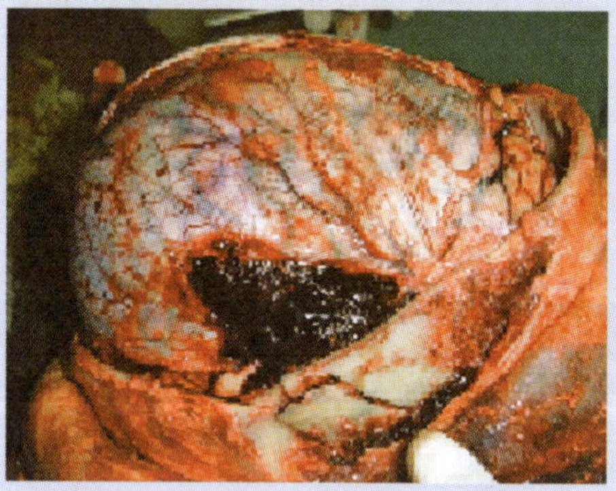

- EDH is usually a COUP INJURY

Clinical features:

- Lucid interval: A period of consciousness between two unconsciousness.

Unconsciousness (due concussion) → Consciousness **Lucid interval** → Unconsciousness (death)

Patient
Can give a valid evidence, valid will and is criminally liable

If patient dies due to medical negligence; the doctor liable under 304A IPC

- Dilated and fixed pupil (due to 3rd cranial nerve palsy) and contralateral hemiparesis.
- **Kernohan's notch phenomenon (ipsilateral hemiparesis, and dilated pupil):**
  - When bleeding increases→ uncal herniation→ impingement on tentorium cerebelli→ compression of fibers of cerebral peduncle→ Kernohan's notch phenomenon
  - False localizing sign.

CT scan: **Biconvex lenticular-shaped**[Q] hemorrhage,

Treatment: It is a surgical emergency, requiring emergency craniotomy and removal of the clot.

Subdural Hemorrhage (SDH)

Types:

- **Aged person** (elderly: More vulnerable even with minor trauma)
- **Rupture of bridging veins**/boxers
- **Child abuse** (Shaken baby syndrome)
    - Bleeding is always from bridging veins or dural venous sinuses.
    - Usually traumatic, following an assault or fall (due to acceleration—deceleration injury)

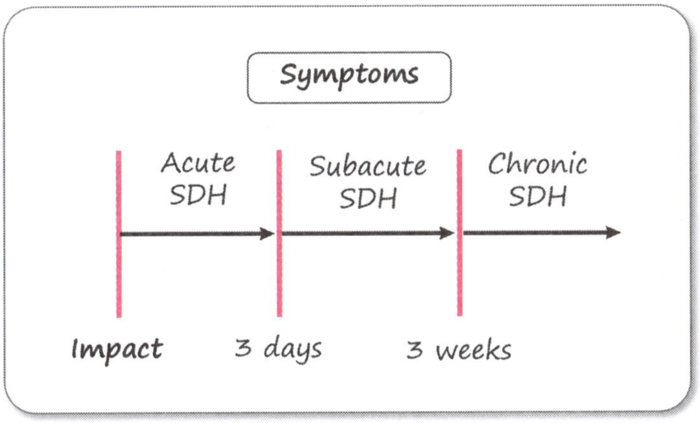

CT scan: Concavo-convex or crescent-shaped[Q] hyperdense collection in subdural space; crossing the suture.

- **Clinical features:**
    - Headache.
    - Altered sensorium.
    - Hemiparesis.
    - Dilated and fixed pupil.
    - Personality changes.
- **Management**
    - Conservative
    - Surgical removal of clot.

Subarachnoid Hemorrhage

Causes

Causes	Clinical features
B – Berry aneurysm rupture A – Arterio venous malformation rupture T – Trauma S – Stroke	**Thunder clap headache**[Q]: Sudden onset of severe headache with vomiting. Features of raised intracranial pressure and Focal neurological deficits: Hemiplegia, dysphasia. Lumbar puncture: **Xanthochromia**[Q] seen. **Surgery:** Clipping/ endovascular coiling of aneurysm

TRANSPORTATION INJURIES

Injuries to Pedestrian

Usual sequence of the impacts with vehicle:

- First, the vehicle hits the person (first impact with vehicle).
- After the first impact, the victim is scooped off the ground and falls on the vehicle (second impact with vehicle).
- Then the victim is thrown on the ground.

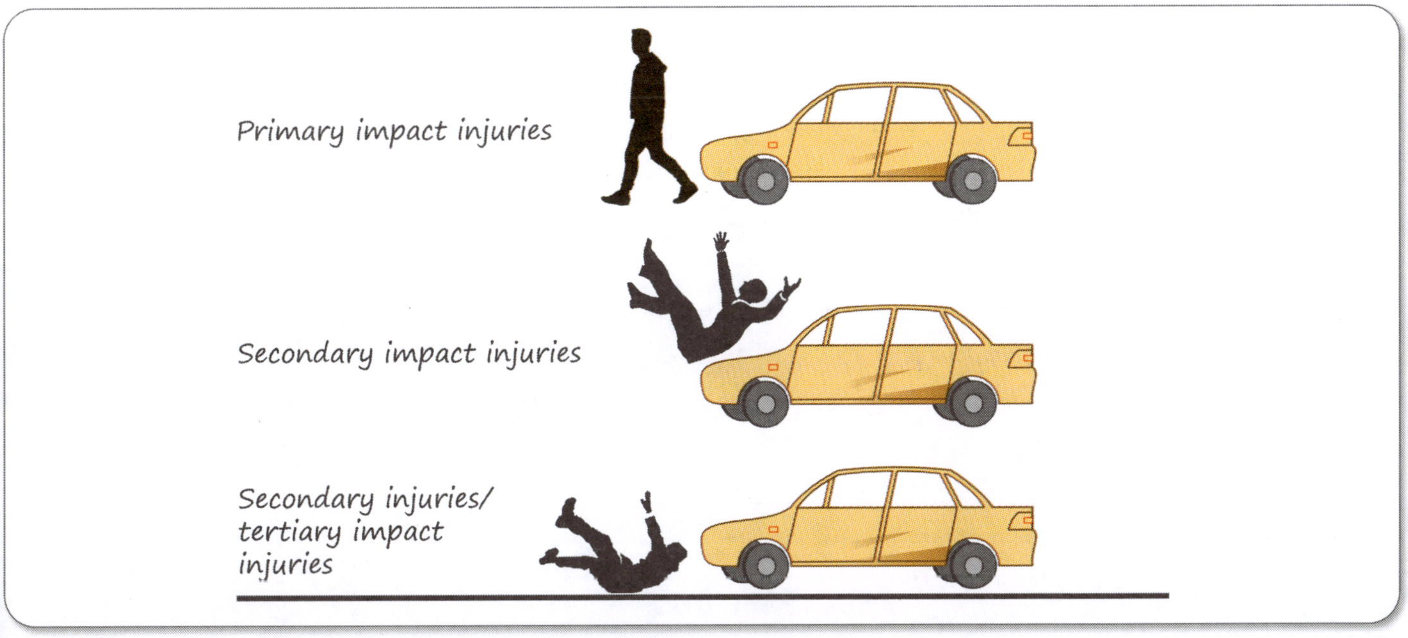

Transportation injuries

- **Primary impact injuries** → 1st site of impact with the vehicle
  - Due to the impact of bumper or radiator
  - Adult-Knee level children-Femur level
  - Bumper injuries present
  - Patterned injuries present
- **Secondary impact injuries** → 2nd impact of victim with the same vehicle
  - Same side of primary impact injuries
  - Severe head injuries present
- **Secondary injuries** → Victim falls on ground
  - Opposite side to primary impact injuries
  - Head injury with brain damage is more common
  - Graze abrasions, bruises and lacerations present

Bumper Injuries

- Primary impact injury[Q].
- Injuries on skin, soft tissues and fracture of bone (bumper fracture).
- The level of bumper injuries varies with the height of bumper in different vehicles.

Bumper Fracture

- Usually in tibia[Q] (sometimes in fibula).
- Triangle[Q] or wedge shaped.
- The base of triangle is the site of impact and the apex of triangle points toward the direction of vehicle.

INJURY TO OCCUPANTS OF A VEHICLE

		Driver	Front seat passenger
Windshield	Multiple cut lacerations on the face—**sparrow foot mark injuries** (due to broken glasses)		
Hyperextension and hyperflexion of neck due to acceleration deceleration trauma.	**Whiplash injury** • Fracture of lower cervical vertebra (C5-C6) • Contusion or laceration of spinal cord without fracture. **Sudden acceleration:** Hyperextension and then flexion. **Sudden deceleration:** Hyperflexion and then extension.	Present	Present
Steering wheel impact	Patterned bruise Fracture of wrist/arm/sternum Aortic rupture	Present	Absent
Seat belt injury	**Direct compression:** Seatbelt bruise/intra abdominal injuries. Deceleration: Most common organ injured: Mesentery Flexion distraction injury: Chance fracture	Present	Present

Contd...

		Driver	Front seat passenger
Dashboard Impact	• Patellar fracture. • Posterior cruciate ligament (PCL) tear. • Posterior dislocation of hip—Dashboard fracture.	Absent	Present

Tail gating[Q] or underrunning:

- The motorcyclist/car driver hits into the back of the heavy vehicle.
- This may be due to unexpected stoppage of the heavy vehicle.
- Head and shoulder injuries, sometimes decapitation.

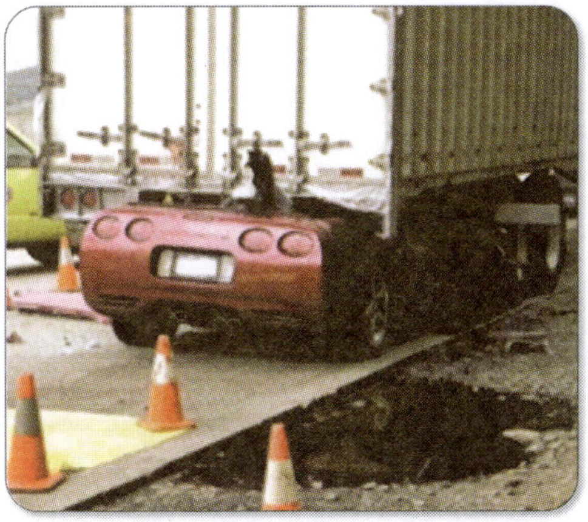

THERMAL INJURIES

Cold injuries		Heat injuries	
General heat	**Local heat**	**General heat**	**Local heat**
Hypothermia	• Frost bite (due to dry cold) • Trench foot (due to moist cold)	• Heat cramps • Heat syncope • Heat stroke	• Burns (due to dry heat) • Scald (due to moist heat[Q])

Hypothermia (Body core temperature less than 35°C)

Common in elderly,alcoholics and newborns.

BCT <32°C = Shivering stops.

Paradoxical undressing:

- May occur in severe hypothermia[Q].
- In terminal stages, the victim becomes disoriented and confused, and may undress himself.
- The body may be found naked or seminaked. There may be suspicion of sexual offence.
- Death is accidental[Q].

Terminal burrowing or Hide-and-Die syndrome:

- Seen in severe hypothermia.
- Victim is often found under bed or bench, behind wardrobe, on a shelf.
- May look like homicide or robbery.

Autopsy findings:

- Pink hypostasis
- Stomach: Wischnewsky spots may be seen.

Frost bite

Due to dry cold exposure (-2.5°C)

Body peripheries involved.

Stages

- **First degree (frostnip):** Pallor
- **Second degree:** Itching and pain followed by numbness
- **Third and fourth degrees:** Painless blisters and necrosis with gangrene formation.

Trench Foot and Immersion Foot

- **Due to moist cold:** Prolonged immersion of foot in water (5°C-8°C)
  Typically seen in soldiers during winter warfare, especially in trenches and in persons exposed to prolonged immersion at sea.
- The extremities are affected in those conditions.

GENERAL HYPERTHERMIA

Disorder	Pathogenesis	Body core temperature	Other features
Heat cramps/Miner's cramps/Fireman's cramps	Electrolyte disturbances due to dehydration.	Normal	
Heat exhaustion/Heat syncope/prostration	**Cardiovascular collapse** and syncope due to intense dehydration	Normal	
Heat stroke Triad of cerebral dysfunction with impaired consciousness, increased body core temperature (rectal) more than 41°C and absence of sweating	**Cerebral dysfunction** Impaired consciousness Absence of sweating except **Exertional heat stroke** **Dry[Q] and hot skin**	>41°C	• Constricted pupils[Q]. • Postmortem caloricity[Q].

BURNS (DUE TO DRY HEAT)

Estimation of affected body surface area:

Area	% of skin burns	
	Rule of nine (adult)	Lund and browder chart (children)
Head	09	18
Upper Limb - L	09	09
Upper Limb - R	09	09
Trunk - Front	18	18
Trunk - Back	18	18
Genitalia	01	01
Lower Limb - L	18	13½
Lower Limb - R	18	13½
TOTAL	100	100

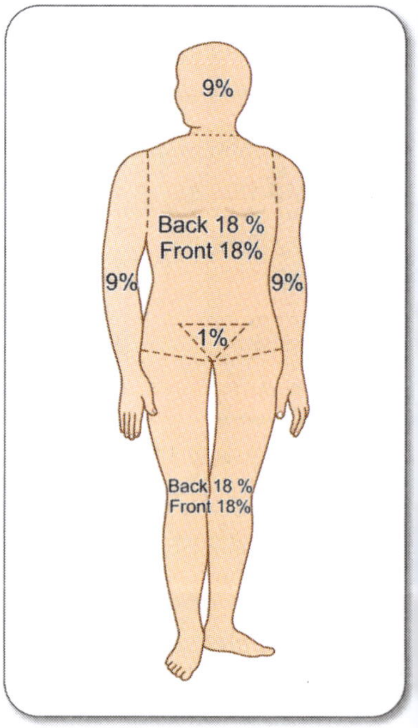

- Involvement of 1/3rd of body surface area (30-50%) is usually fatal.

Rule of palms:
- For estimating small burns[Q].
- The surface area of a patient's palm (including fingers) = **1% of TBSA**[Q].

- **For burns in adults:** 'Rule of Wallace' or 'Rule of nine.'
- **For burns in children:** 'Lund and browder chart.'
- **For patchy burns:** 'Rule of palm.'

Autopsy Findings

Heat artefacts (nonspecific signs)

Heat stiffening	Heat rupture	Heat hematoma	Heat fracture
Due to coagulation of muscle proteins[Q].	Skin splits occurring due to severe burning[Q]. • **Sites:** Fleshy areas, extensor surfaces and joints. • Resembles incised or lacerated wounds[Q].	**Heat exposure to head—emissary veins/dural venous sinus rupture → Clot in extradural space** • **Resembles traumatic extradural hematoma**	**Skull fractures** • Usually seen on either side above the temples. • Usually stellate. **Long bone fracture** • Due to excessive shrinkage of the muscles, which exert great pull on bones. • **Street and avenue fracture**
Pugilistic attitude (boxing, fencing or defense attitude/ heat stiffening)	Multiple and large (several centimeters) **Floor: Intact vessels** **Pale, no bleeding**	• Bilateral and diffuse. • Honeycomb appearance. • Chocolate brown clot. • Presence of carboxyhemoglobin (CoHb) in clot.	

Specific Findings of Antemortem Burns

External (mnemonic FIRE)	Internal
F – Fluid in blisters I – Inflammatory reaction in burns R – Redness (erythema)/red line around burns and blisters E – Elevated enzymes in the positive zone of burns	C – Carbon (soot) deposition in the airway. C – CoHb elevated in blood C – Cyanide level elevated in blood C – Curling's ulcer

Note: Carbon and soot particles in larynx, trachea and bronchioles—**most certain sign of antemortem burns[Q].**

How to differentiate antemortem from postmortem blisters?

Antemortem vesicles	Postmortem vesicles
• **Content:** Serous fluid containing albumin and chlorides. • The base is inflamed and red with erythematous borders[Q].	• **Content:** Gas[Q]. • The base is dry, hard and yellow.

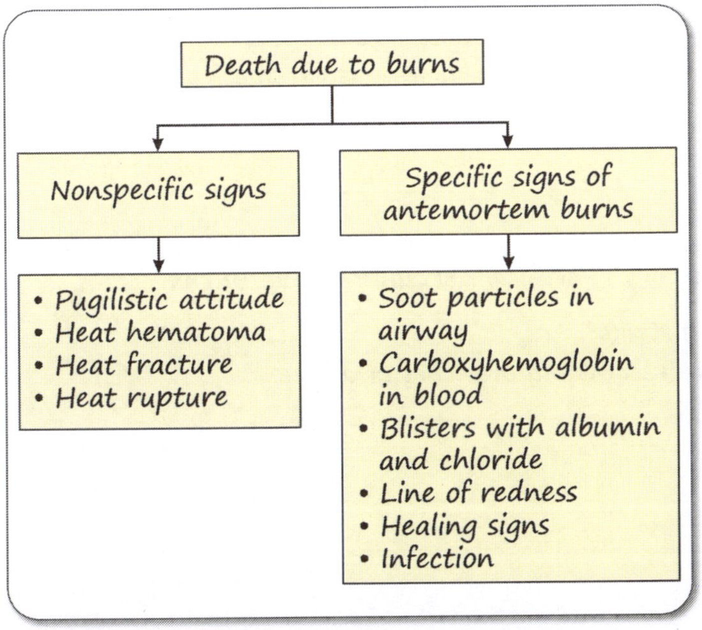

SCALDS

- Injury caused by moist heat; liquids above 60°C
- Injury at and below the site of contact.
- Maximum damage at the point of commencement.
- Restricted to exposed body parts or point of contact.
- No charring, carbonization or hair singeing[Q] in scalds.
- Evidence of splashing present.
- Skin sodden and bleached[Q].
- Blisters over the burnt area.

ELECTROCUTION INJURIES

Alternating current (AC) is 4–5 times more dangerous than direct current (DC).

Current (Amperes) Most important factor to determine fatality.	Voltage	Resistance
• 5 mA—numbness, pain. • 10–15 mA—tetany within the flexor muscles of hand and forearm • 40 mA—ventricular arrhythmia • >50 mA—instantly fatal.	When voltage increases, the chances of injury increases.	The principal bodily barrier is the skin. Dry skin offers high resistance (1000–1500 Ohm), but resistance in wet skin is only 200–300 Ohm.

Causes of Death (Depends on the Path of Current)

- Ventricular fibrillation[Q]—most common cause.
- Respiratory failure

Effects of Electrocution

Joule burns[Q]: Firm contact with low voltage current	**Spark burn**[Q]: Loose contact with air gap.
Endogenous burn[Q] • Joule burns, also known as electrical burns are **specific**[Q] **and diagnostic of electric burns** • Round, shallow, pale central crater, with a raised border around. • Joule burn is commonly found on palmar aspects of hands. **Metallization of entry wound:** Deposition of metallic ions from conductor in entry wound (detected by **Acro reaction test**)	**Crocodile burns:** Loose contact with High voltage current. Multiple punched out spark lesions over the exposed parts of the body due to arcing of high tension current[Q]. **Current pearls:** • Deposition of molten metal from the conductor into the tissues. • Identified by scanning electron microscopy. **Bone pearls:** • Heat generated by the current may melt the calcium phosphate in bone. • Radiographically seen as rarefactive foci in X-ray limbs.

LIGHTNING INJURIES

Arborescent Burns/Filigree Burns[Q]/Lichtenberg's Flowers[Q]/Ferning/Keraunographic Burns

- Lichtenberg flowers are **pathognomonic of lightning strike**[Q].
- Superficial thin irregular tortuous markings on skin resembling branches of a tree.
- Does not correspond to vascular channels.
- Found over shoulders or flanks.

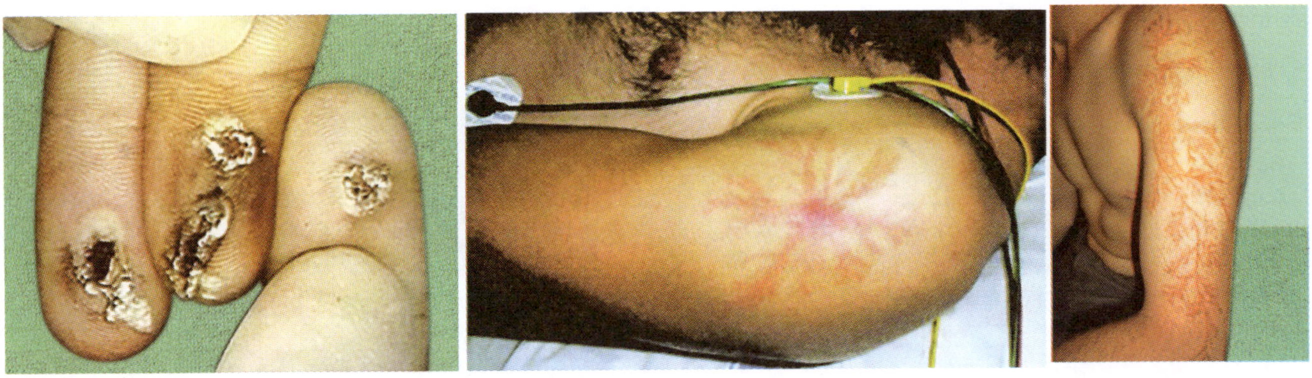

EXPLOSION INJURIES: INJURIES PRODUCED BY BOMB EXPLOSION

A bomb is a container filled with an explosive mixture and missiles, which is fired either by detonator or a fuse.

Types Blast Injuries

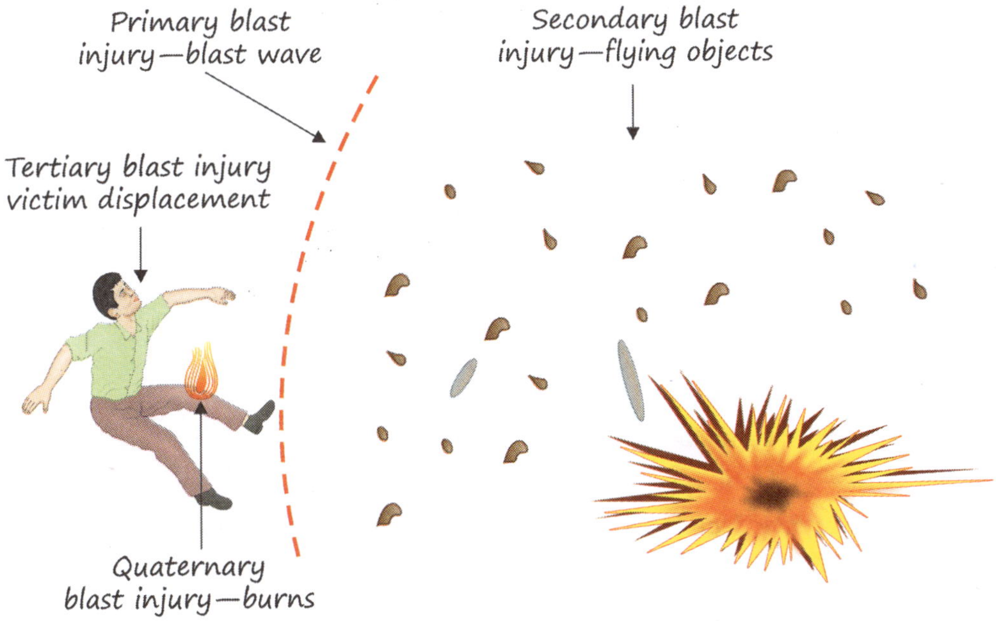

Primary blast injuries	Blast wave[Q]
Secondary blast injuries	Flying projectiles[Q]
Tertiary blast injuries	Victim displacement[Q]
Quaternary blast injuries	Structural collapse/fire[Q]
Quinary blast injuries	Hyperinflammatory state due to chemical/radiation

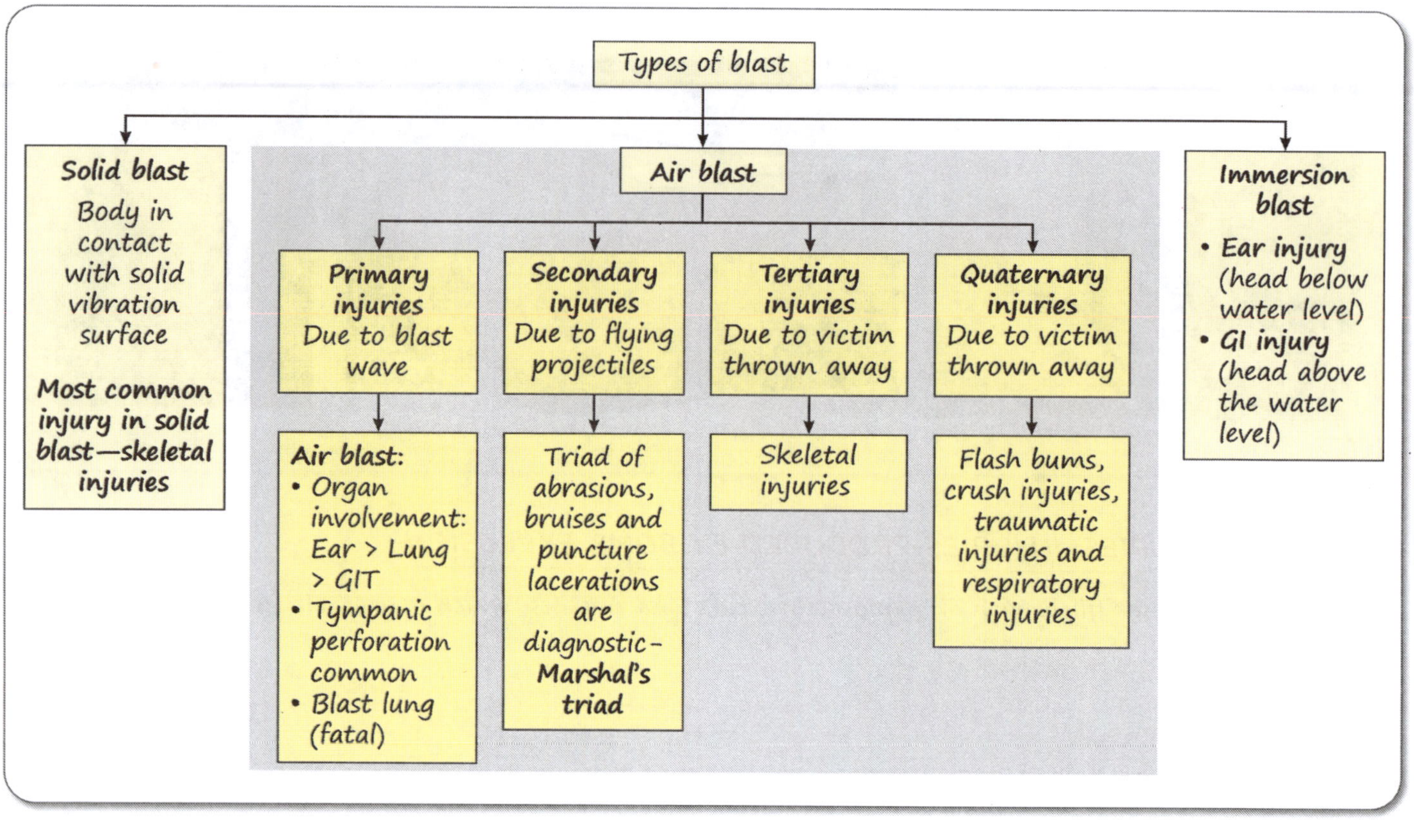

Order of organ involvement in primary blast injuries:
- ***In air:*** *Tympanic membrane, lung and GIT*
- *Under water (head above water level): GIT, lung and ear*
- *Under water (head under water level): Ear, GIT and lung.*

TORTURE METHODS

Falanga (bastinado)[Q]	Beating over the soles.
Telefono[Q]	Repeated slapping over ears.
Wet submarine[Q]	Forced immersion of head in water.
Dry submarine[Q]	Tying a plastic bag over the head.
Parrot's perch	Head down from a horizontal pole placed under the knees with wrists bound to ankle.
Cattle prod	Electric shock, especially over the genitals.
Dunking	Victim is immersed into water, taken out after some time and given a chance to confess.
Black slave	Heated metal skewer inserted into the anus.
El planton	Prolonged standing.
Saw horse	Forced straddling of a bar.

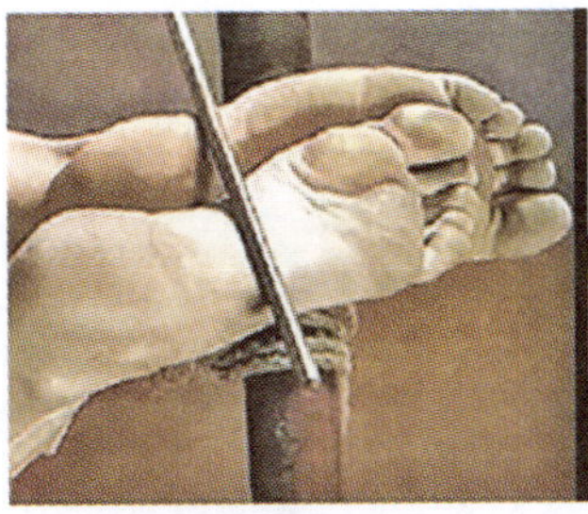
Falanga

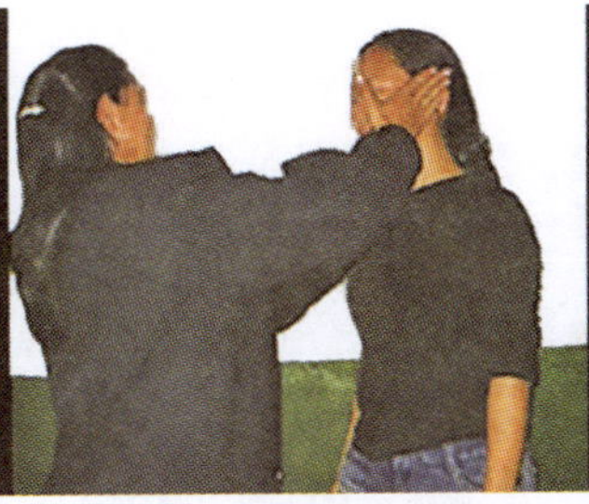
Telefono

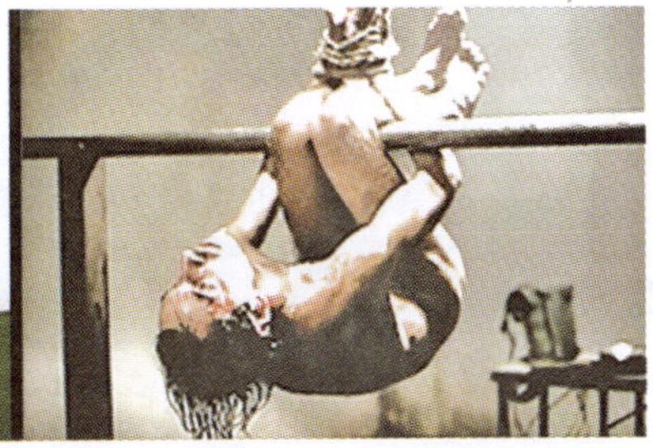
Parrot perch

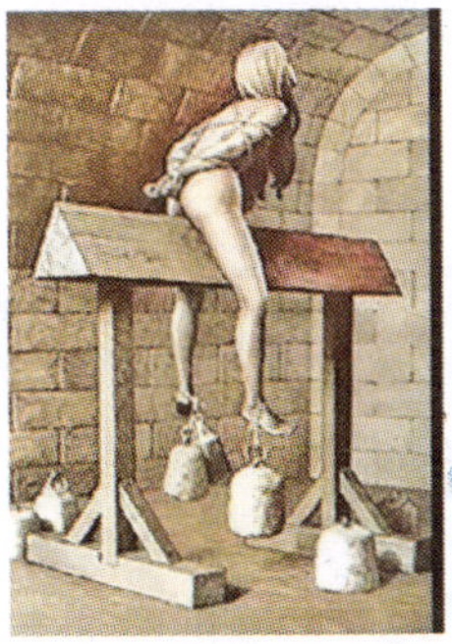
Saw horse

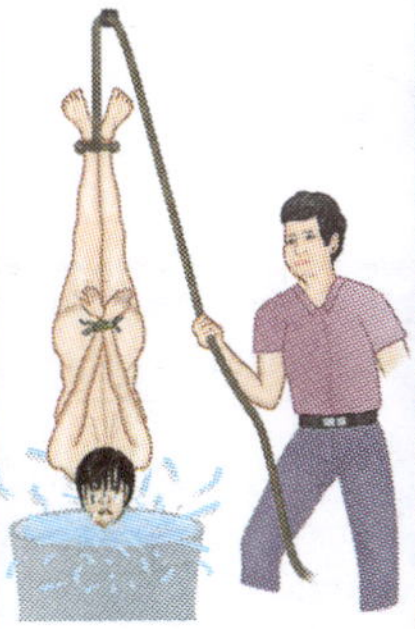
Wet submarine

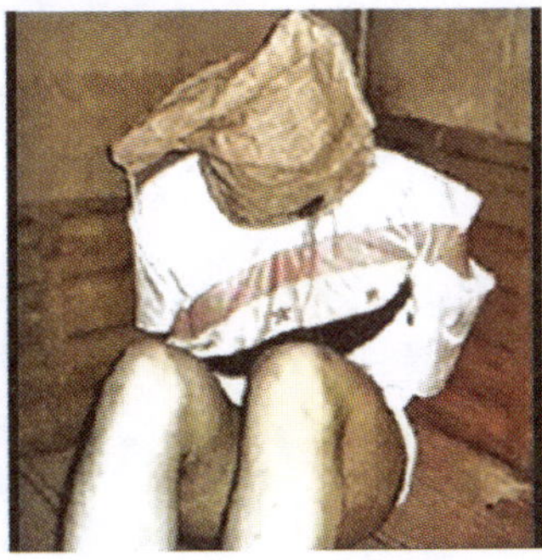
Dry submarine

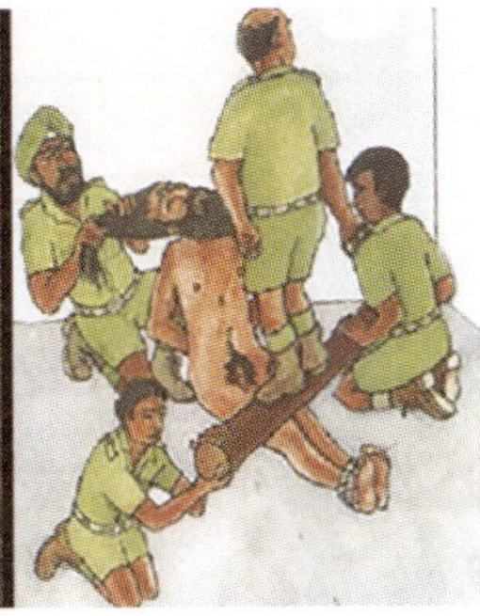
Ghotna

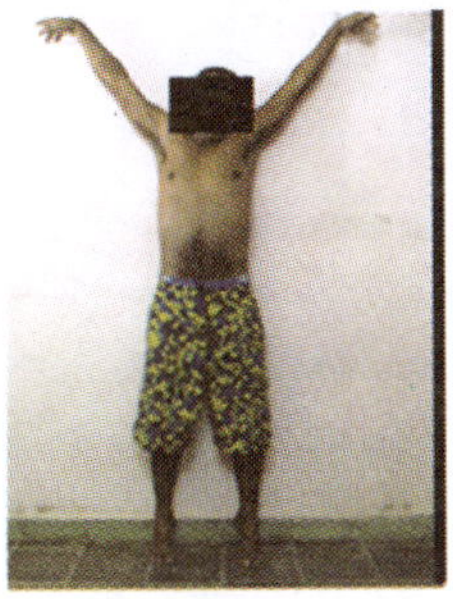
EL planton

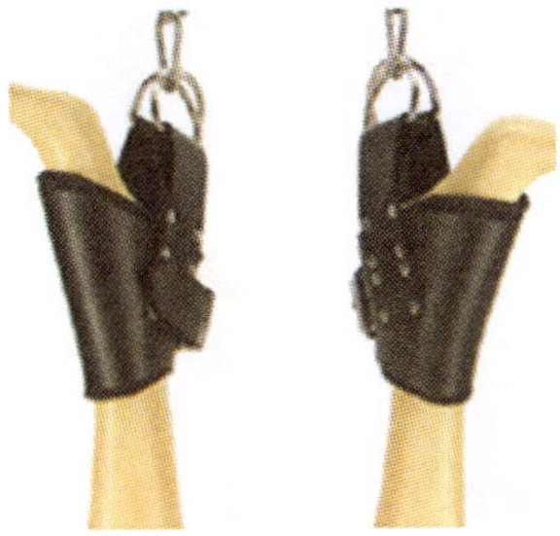
Mercelago

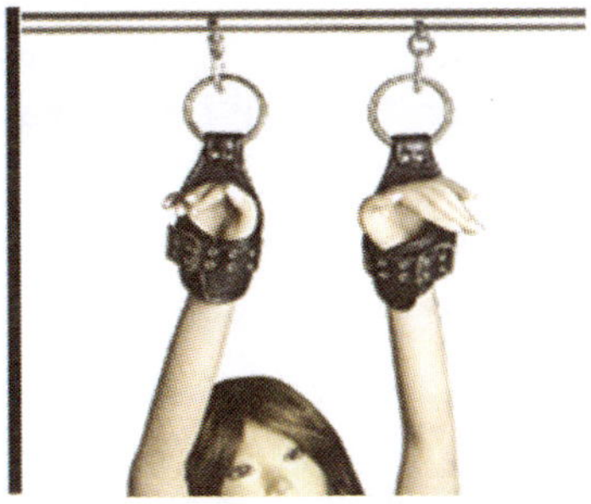
LA bandera

FORENSIC BALLISTICS

- **Internal or proximal ballistics:** Study of the projectile within the gun.
- **External or intermediate ballistics:** Study of the passage of the projectile through the air.
- **Wound or terminal ballistics:** Study of the effects of projectile on the tissues.

Basic Structure of a Firearm

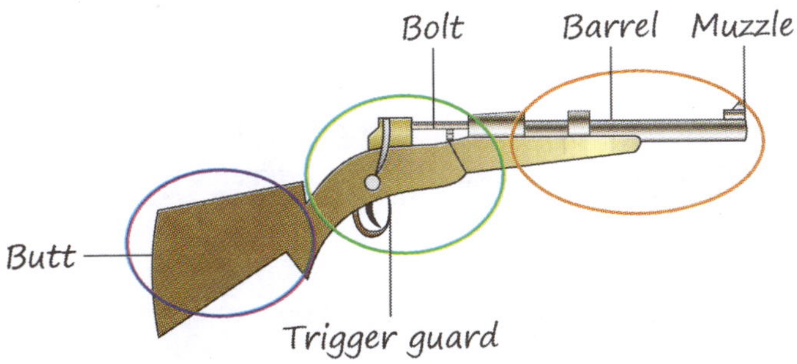

Classification of Firearm

Firearms can be broadly classified into Rifled firearms and smooth bore firearms.

Rifled gun Projectiles: BULLET	Smooth bore gun Projectile: LEAD SHOTS/LEAD PELLETS
Any gun having grooves (rifling) in the bore is called rifled gun. 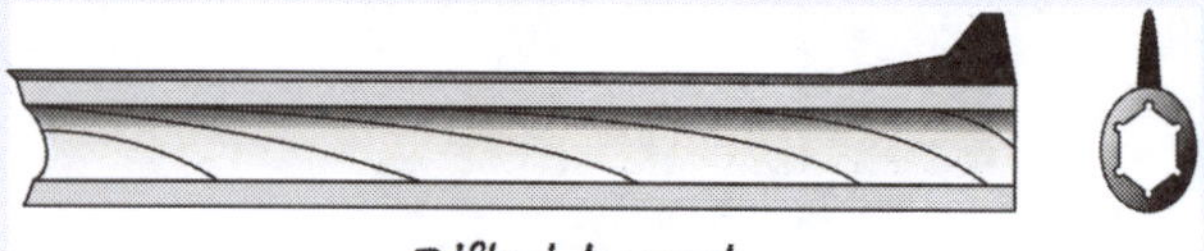 Rifled barrel Example: • Rifles: 0.22, single shot, lever action, bolt action • Revolvers, pistols	The bore is uniformly smooth without any grooves in shot gun. 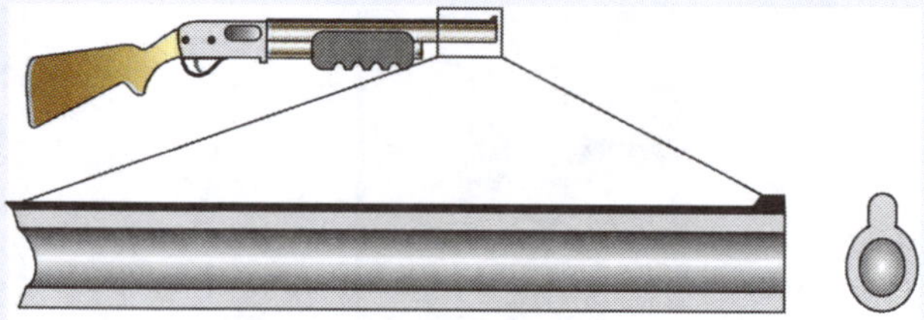 Typical shotgun barrel
Rifling The interior of barrel, i.e., bore has 4–6 grooves running parallel to each other from breech end to muzzle end. The elevated areas are called lands and depressed areas are called grooves. 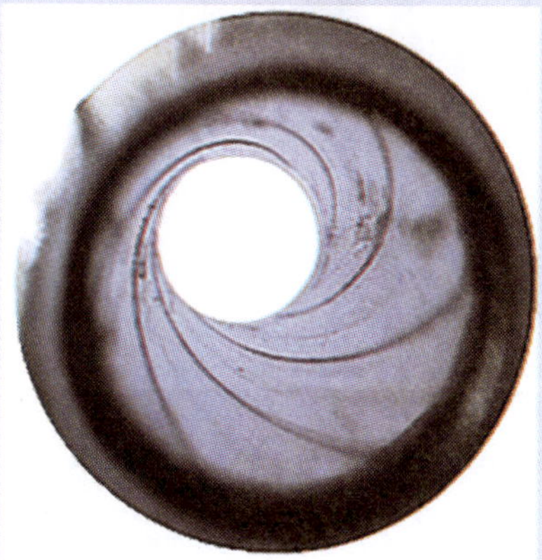 **Advantages of rifling:** • Imparts spinning motion[Q] to the bullet. • Straight trajectory. • Prevents wobbling of bullets.	**Choking:** In shotgun, the distal 10 cm of barrel is constricted. 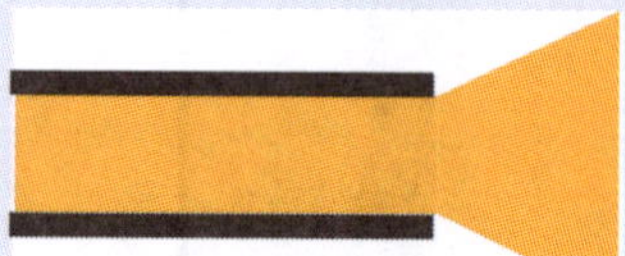 Unchoked 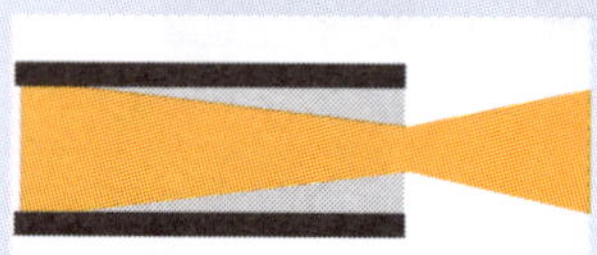 Full choked **Advantages of choking in shot gun:** • Reduces the pellets dispersion[Q]. • Increases the explosive forces of the pellets. **Depending on choking:** • Unchoked or cylinder bore **(maximum dispersion[Q])**. • Quarter choked. • Half choked. • Fully choked **(least dispersion)**.

- **Paradox guns:** If the barrel is partly smooth bored and partly rifled.
- **Helixometer:** Instrument to examine the interior of the barrel.

Bore/Calibre/Gauge:
It is measured by the internal dimension of the barrel

Rifled gun calibre

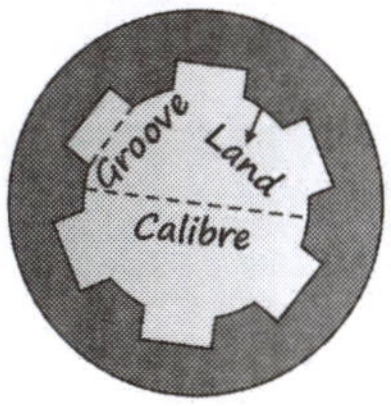

- It is the diameter of the interior of the barrel of **a rifled gun**
- **Measured between diagonally opposite lands**
- Expressed in inches or millimeters, e.g. .22", .32", .38"

Smooth bore gun caliber

For small bores:
Direct method:
The internal diameter of the barrel

For large bores:
Indirect method:

1 Pound (454 g) of lead taken

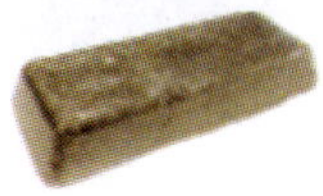

Lead balls are mode.
Size of the lead ball = size of the barrel

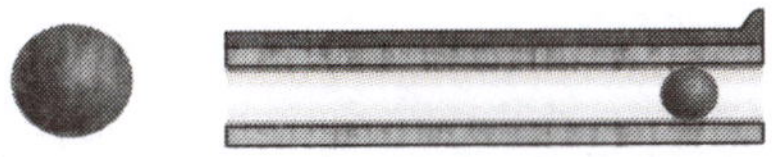

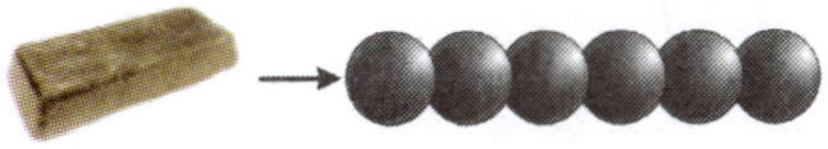

The number of equally sized lead balls made from 1 pound of lead = Gauge

Bore = Number of spherical lead balls taken to fill the barrel.
For example, 12 bore gun – 12 lead balls are made from 1 pound lead
24 bore gun-24 lead balls are made from 1 pound lead

Structure of Ammunition

Constituents of shotgun cartridge (from base to top)	Constituents of rifled gun-bullet (from base to top)
(Detonator cap) percussion cap containing primer mixture	(Detonator cap) percussion cap containing primer mixture
Gun powder	Gun powder
Thick felt-wad	Bullet
Lead shots	
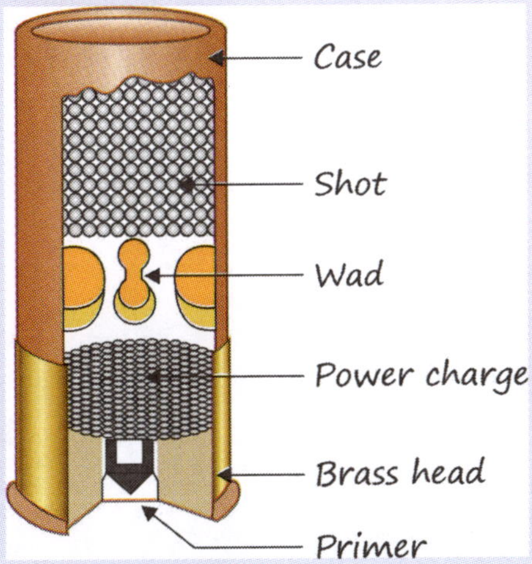	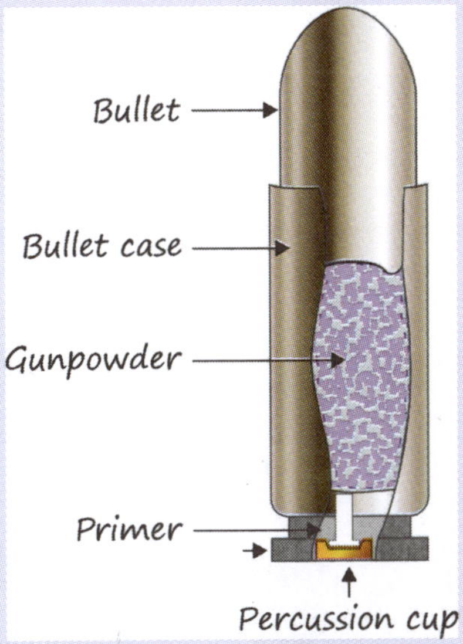

Percussion Chamber/Primer Cup/Detonator cap

- Percussion chamber it contains the priming mixture[Q].
- The strike of firing pin on the primer cup ignites the priming mixture and burns it.
- The fire flashes through the flash hole/vent and ignites the gun powder.

Gun Powder

Black gun powder	Smokeless gun powder	Semi smokeless gun powder
Smoke: More Energy: 3–4 L gas/g • Described as FG, FFG, FFFG, FFFFG depending on the fineness of the grain[Q]. • The finer grains have more number of 'F'	Smoke: Less Energy: 12–13 L gas/g • Single base: Nitrocellulose • Double base: Nitrocellulose + Nitroglycrine[Q] • Triple base: Nitrocellulose + Nitroglycerine + Nitroguanidine	
Potassium nitrate 75% Charcoal 15% Sulphur 10%	Nitrocellulose Nitroglycerine Nitroguanidine	Black gun powder (80%) + Smokeless (20%)

Constituents of Primer

B – Barium nitrate
L - Lead peroxide
A – Antimony
S – Styphnate (lead styphnate)
T – Tetrazine

Working Mechanism of Firearm

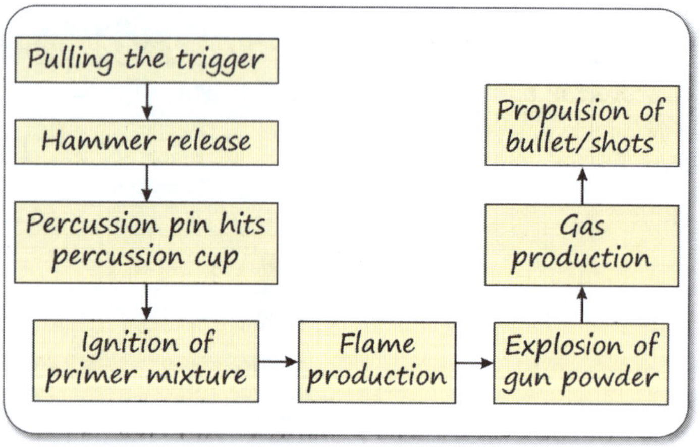

Effects of Discharges of a Gun

- **Fire/flame:** Burning at entrance wound along with burning or singeing of hairs.
- **Smoke:** Blackening effect or smudging.
- **Unburnt gun powder**: Tattooing effect, peppering or stippling effect.
- **Felt wad:** Minor abrasion and bruise.
- **Bullet: Punctured wound**
  - Grease collar/dirt collar/**bullet wipe**[Q]
  - Abrasion collar

Abrasion Collar/Ring: A rim of abraded skin around entry wound.

In rifled gun entrance wounds[Q].

Mechanism: The skin around the entry wound is abraded due to the spinning action of bullet.

Importance

Round abrasion collar[Q]: If bullet hits at right angle to the skin surface.

Oval abrasion collar[Q]: If bullet hits at oblique angle to the skin surface.

Grease Collar (Bullet Wipe): Due to the deposition of lubricants, gun oil or lead from the bullet.

Abrasion collar surrounds the dirt collar.

Dirt collar rim is more prominent in clothing—'bullet wipe'.

Dirt collars are proof of an entry wound.

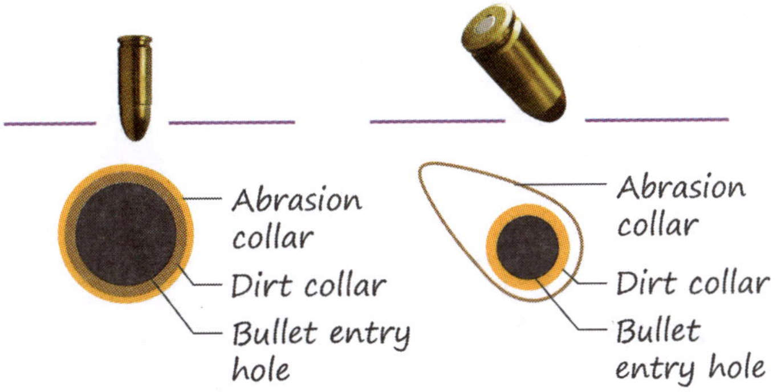

WOUND BALLISTICS

Rifled Gun Injuries

Contact	Contact with skin
Close	Inside the flame
Near	Outside flame, inside the smoke
Intermediate	Outside smoke, inside gun powder
Distant	Outside gun powder

Specific appearances of contact shot

Muzzle/recoil imprint abrasion:

- Patterned abrasion caused by the expansive power of the gases lifting the skin forcibly up against the muzzle.

Back spatter:

- In a contact shot, negative pressure in the barrel may suck blood, hair, tissue fragments back into the barrel.

Blowback phenomenon[Q] or blast effect[Q]:

- Cruciate, stellate or ragged laceration is seen, especially if there is a bone under the skin (skull).

Contact Shot:

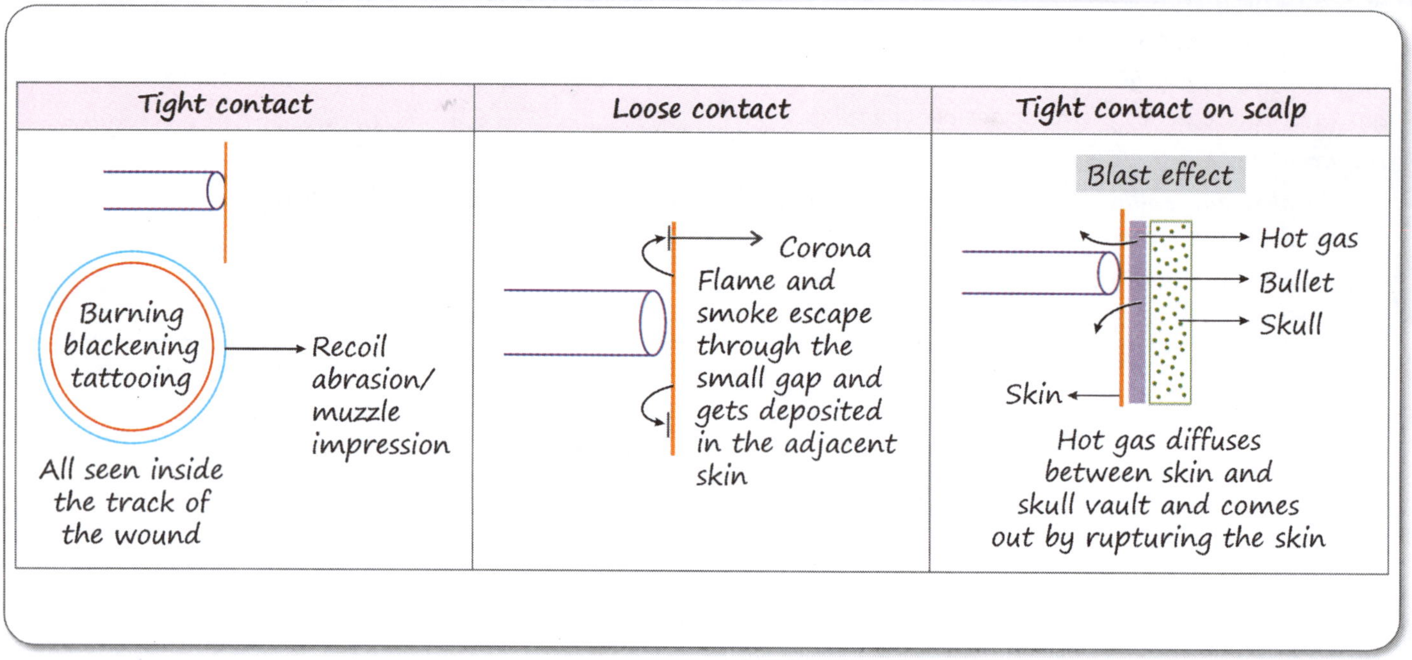

Appearance of Wound of Rifled Firearm in Different Ranges

Close shot (range of flame)	Near range (outside the flame inside the smoke)	Intermediate range (outside smoke inside the gunpowder)	Long range (outside gun powder)[Q]
• Circular entrance wound	• Circular entrance wound	• Circular entrance wound	• Circular wound smaller than the diameter of the bullet
• Burns and singeing—Present • Blackening[Q]—Present	• Burning/blackening—present • Tattooing[Q]—Present	• Burning/blackening—absent • Tattooing[Q]—present	• Burning, blackening tattooing—Absent
• Tattooing—Present • Punctured wound/ grease collar/ abrasion collar—present	• Punctured wound/ grease collar/ abrasion collar—present	• Punctured wound/ grease collar/ abrasion collar—present	• Punctured wound/ grease collar/ abrasion collar—present
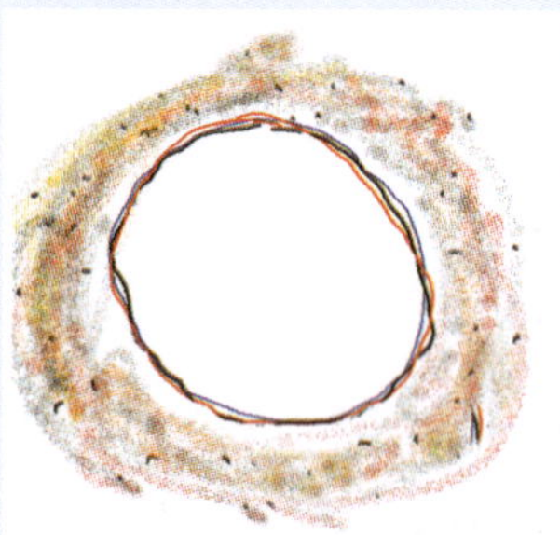	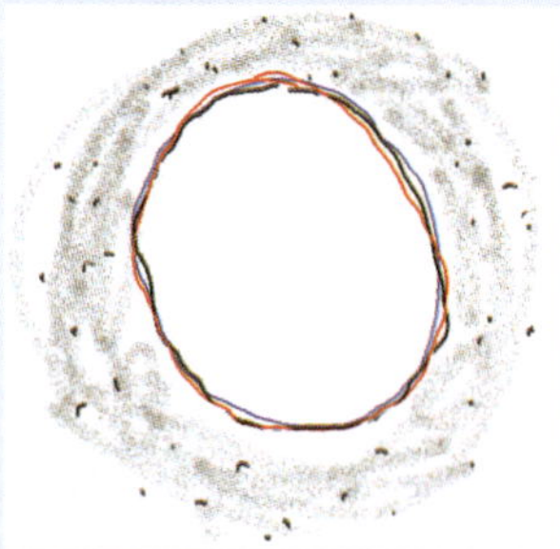	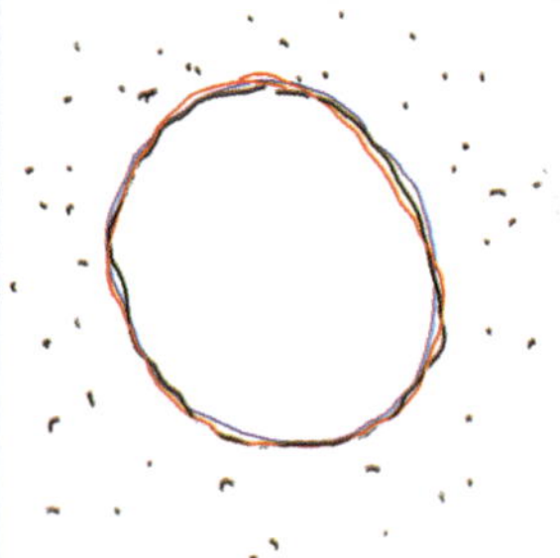	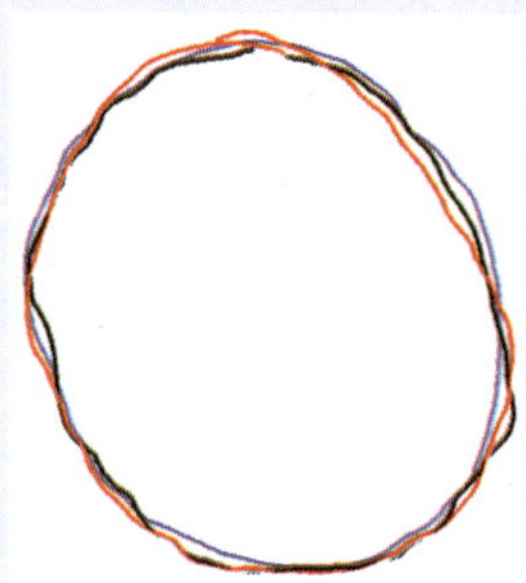

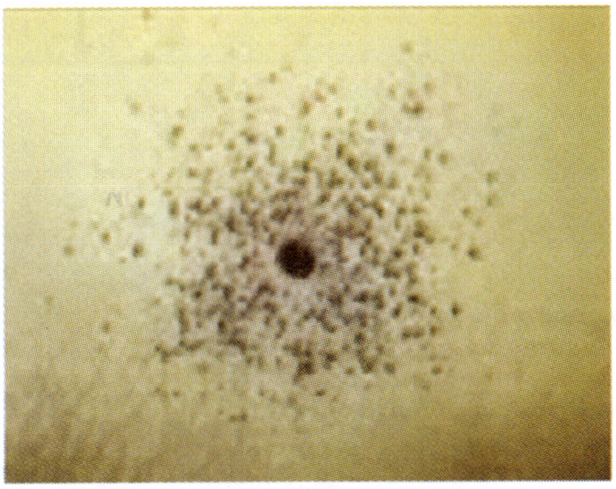

Intermediate shot

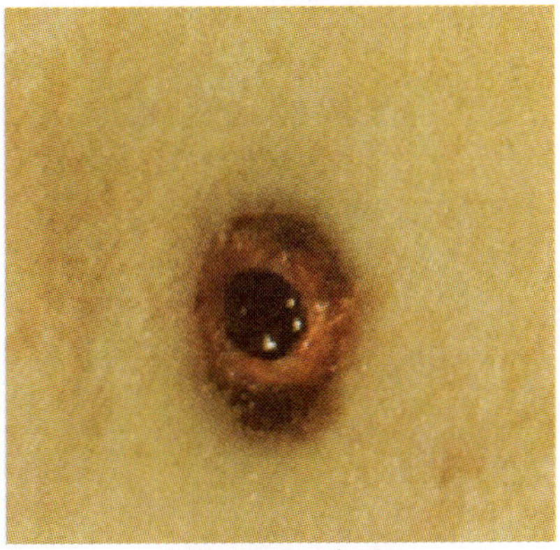

Distant shot

Shot gun injuries: In shot gun, there is dispersion of lead shots.

Definition of ranges in shot gun:

- **Contact range:** Muzzle end of gun is in tight contact with skin.
- **Close range:** <1 m
- **Near range:** 1–2 m
- **Intermediate range:** 2–4 m
- **Distant range:** >4 m

Effects of flame, smoke, tattooing are noted within 1 m. (beyond 1 m, only lead shot injuries seen)

Dispersion of lead shots starts at 2 m; complete dispersion is seen at 4 m[Q]

Important points to remember:

- **Effects of flame, smoke, tattooing are noted within 1 m. (beyond 1 m, only lead shot injuries seen)** Burns, blackening and tattooing around entrance wound till 1 m.
- **Dispersion of lead shots start at 2 m; complete dispersion is seen at 4 m**[Q]
  - All the lead shots enter the skin as single mass till 2 m.
    - After 2 m, lead shots begin to disperse and individual pellet holes can be found in addition to central big hole.
    - At 4 m, there is complete dispersion of lead shots and only individual pellet holes are seen.

Appearance of Wound of Shot Gun in Different Ranges

The appearance of contact shot is similar to the contact shot of rifled gun namely, tight skin contact, loose skin contact and contact on bony prominence.

Close range (<1 m)	Near range (1–2 m)	Intermediate range (2–4 m)	Distant range (>4 m)
• Single circular entrance wound • **Burns/singeing—Present** • **Blackening—present** • **Tattooing—present**	• Single entrance wound • Irregular margins **—Rat hole appearance**[Q]	• Central hole due to shot mass surrounded by individual pellet hole • As the distance increases from 2 to 4 m, the size of central hole decreases and the pellet dispersion increases	**Individual pellet holes** due to complete dispersion

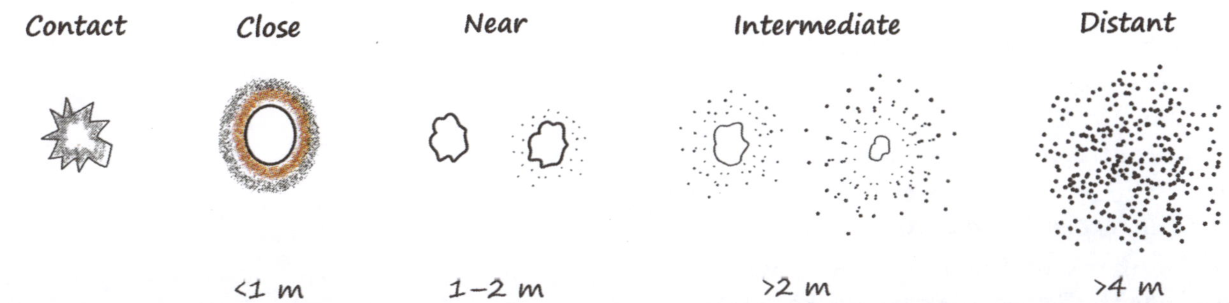

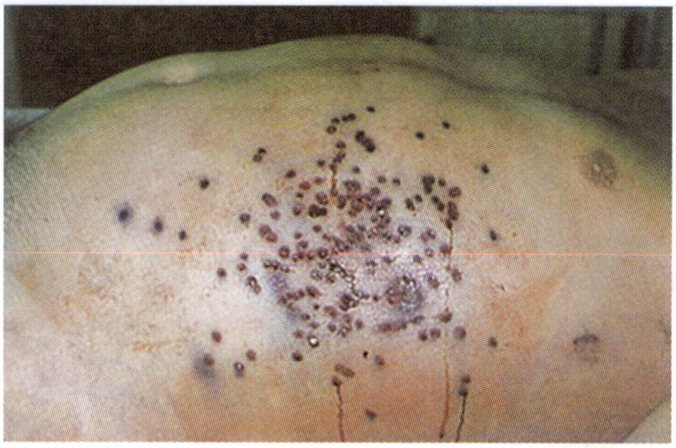

Entry Wound versus Exit Wounds

Character	Entry wound	Exit wound
Size	Smaller than the diameter of the bullet	Larger
Edges	Inverted	Everted[Q]
Abrasion collar and grease collar	Present[Q]	Absent[Q]
Scorching, smudging and tattooing	May be present	Absent
Bleeding	Less	More[Q]
Fat extrusion	Absent	May be present
Cherry red color	May be present	Absent

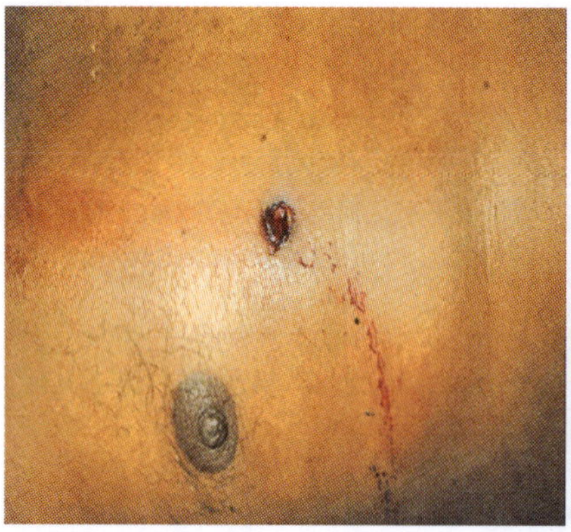

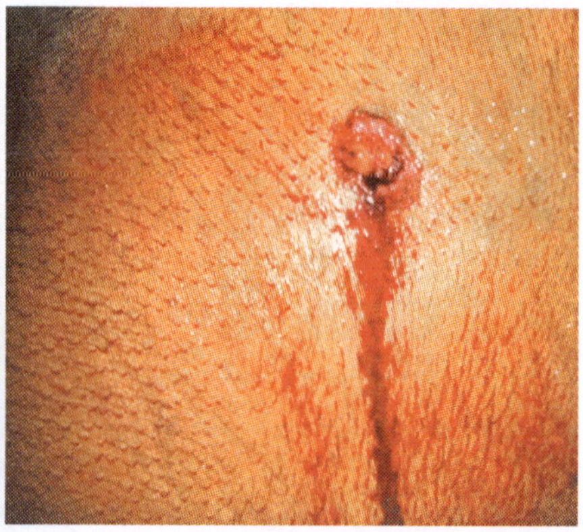

How to find out whether the recovered bullet has been fired from the alleged firearm?

Bullet finger printing: Technique of identifying the gun from the bullet markings.

Two types of markings:

Primary marking/class characteristics: Due to rifling grooves of barrel[Q] (macroscopic).

- Every gun model has specific rifling pattern.
- Primary markings are used to identify the make and model of the guns involved.

Secondary Markings or Individual/Accidental Characteristics

- Imperfections produced accidentally during the manufacturing or due to sticking of lead particles to the bore when shots are fired (metallic fouling)
- Secondary Markings produced on bullet surface by such imperfections[Q] (microscopic)

They are useful in identifying the specific gun which was fired **(fingerprint of a gun)**

Study of comparison of markings on crime bullet and test bullet under comparison microscope—**Bullet finger printing**[Q]

How to find out WHO HAS FIRED THE GUN? whether the recovered bullet has been fired from the alleged firearm?

GSR test (Detection of gunshot residue)

H - Harrison and Gilroy

A - Atomic absorption spectrometry (AAS)

N - Neutron activation analysis

D - Dermal nitrate test

S - SEM-EDXA (most specific)

Swabs taken from the hand dorsum and palms

Mnemonic: **HANDS**

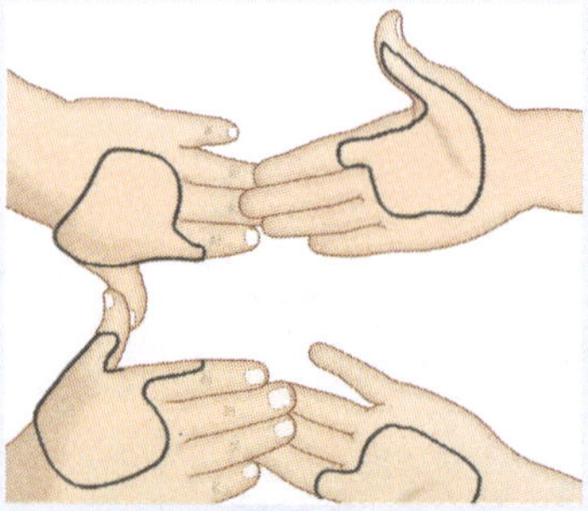

To elicit GSR in clothing: Infrared photography.

Puppe's Rule

- For skull injuries due to **multiple impacts**Q. (gunshot/blunt impact)
- **The sequence of impacts**Q can be established.

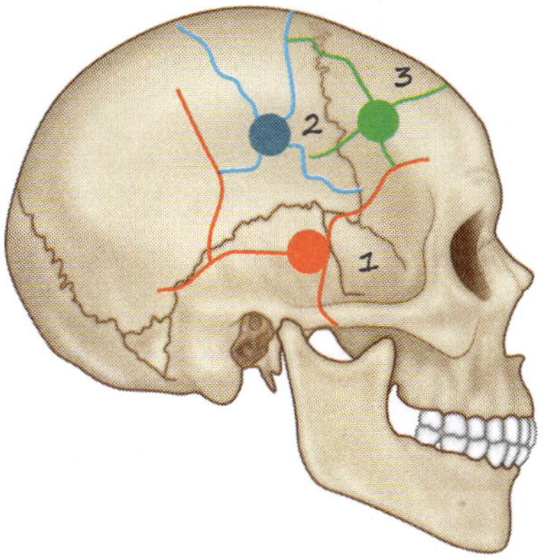

- When there are two fracture lines in the skull, the second fracture will always be stopped by the preexisting fracture line.

Gunshot Wounds on Skull

Principle

Skull has outer table and inner table.

When the bullet enters the skull tables, bevelling occurs in the **unsupported table** (second layer).

	Entrance wound	Exit wound
Skull outer table	Clean cut hole	Bevelled openingQ
Skull Inner table	Bevelled openingQ	Clean cut hole

ATYPICAL BULLETS

Tandem Bullet/Piggyback Bullet

- Seen with old unused gun/faulty ammunition.
- **Two bullets**Q come out of the muzzle end.

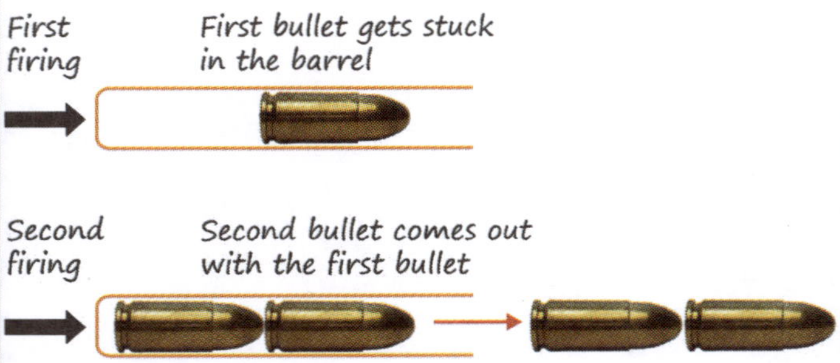

Dum Dum Bullet/Mushrooming Bullet/**Semi Jacketed bullet**Q

- When Dum Dum bullet enters/strikes the skin, it expands like a mushroom and produces more damage.

Frangible Bullet (Made of Powdered Iron/Copper)

- Gets fragmented on impact, for limited penetration.
- Impact can cause lead snowstorm.

Tracer Bullet

Tracer bullet leaves a **visible mark or 'trace' while in flight**Q, so that the path of bullet can be seen.

Incendiary Bullets

- Incendiary bullets contain **phosphorus**Q at the tip.
- Type of army bullet used to cause fire in the target.

Yawning Bullet

- A bullet traveling in an irregular fashion instead of traveling nose-onQ is called a yawning bullet.
- May cause key hole entry woundQ.

Tumbling Bullet

Tumbling bullet that rotates end-on-end during its motionQ

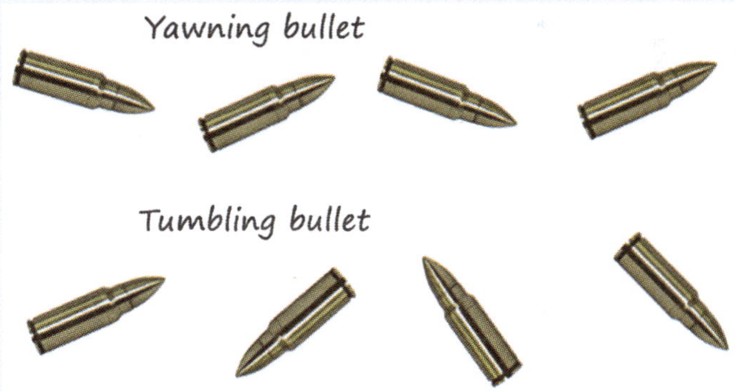

Ricochet Bullet (Deflected Bullet)

Bullet **strikes some intervening object first**Q, and then after ricocheting, hits the victim.

After Ricocheting

- No burning, blackening and tattooing seen.
- **Abrasion collar is absent**Q, as the bullet loses its spinning motion.
- The entry wound may be atypical, as the **bullet may be deformed**.

Souvenir Bullets

Retained bullet[Q] inside the body for a long time

- Dense fibrous tissue surrounds the bullet.
- Chronic lead poisoning may occur due to absorption of lead from the bullet into the body fluids.

Plastic Bullets or Baton Round

Made up of polyvinyl chloride.

Kennedy Phenomenon

- **Iatrogenic surgical alteration[Q]** of the entrance wound.
- The evaluation of whether the wound is entrance or exit becomes difficult.

Rayalaseema Phenomenon

- Rayalaseema phenomenon is an artifact.
- A bullet is implanted in a stab injury to fake a firearm injury.
- It is done to mislead the investigations.

ATYPICAL APPEARANCES IN SHOTGUN WOUNDS

Billiard ball ricochet effect	Balling or welding of shot
• When the lead shots pass through an intermediate object like glass or the body part is covered with a thick jacket, the lead shots face momentary resistance and they strike each other. • It results in wide spread dispersion of lead shots in the entry wound. • Such wide dispersion of lead shots may suggest a long range fire (even though actually it is close range fire).	• Cause: Faulty manufacture or Pouring of paraffin wax into the cartridge. • Some lead shots, ball together to form a compact mass. • The balled shots and the remaining dispersed lead shots enter the skin separately. • Such appearance may suggest a intermediate range fire (even though actually it is a distant range fire).

5. FORENSIC TOXICOLOGY

- Father of toxicology: Paracelsus.
- Father of modern toxicology: Mathieu orifila.
- Poison: Any substance given in any form, any route (oral, injectable, inhalation, contact) causing ill health or death by its local or remote action.
- Rapid onset: Inhalation > IV > IM.
- According to paracelsus, 'the dose makes the poison'.

CLASSIFICATION OF POISONS

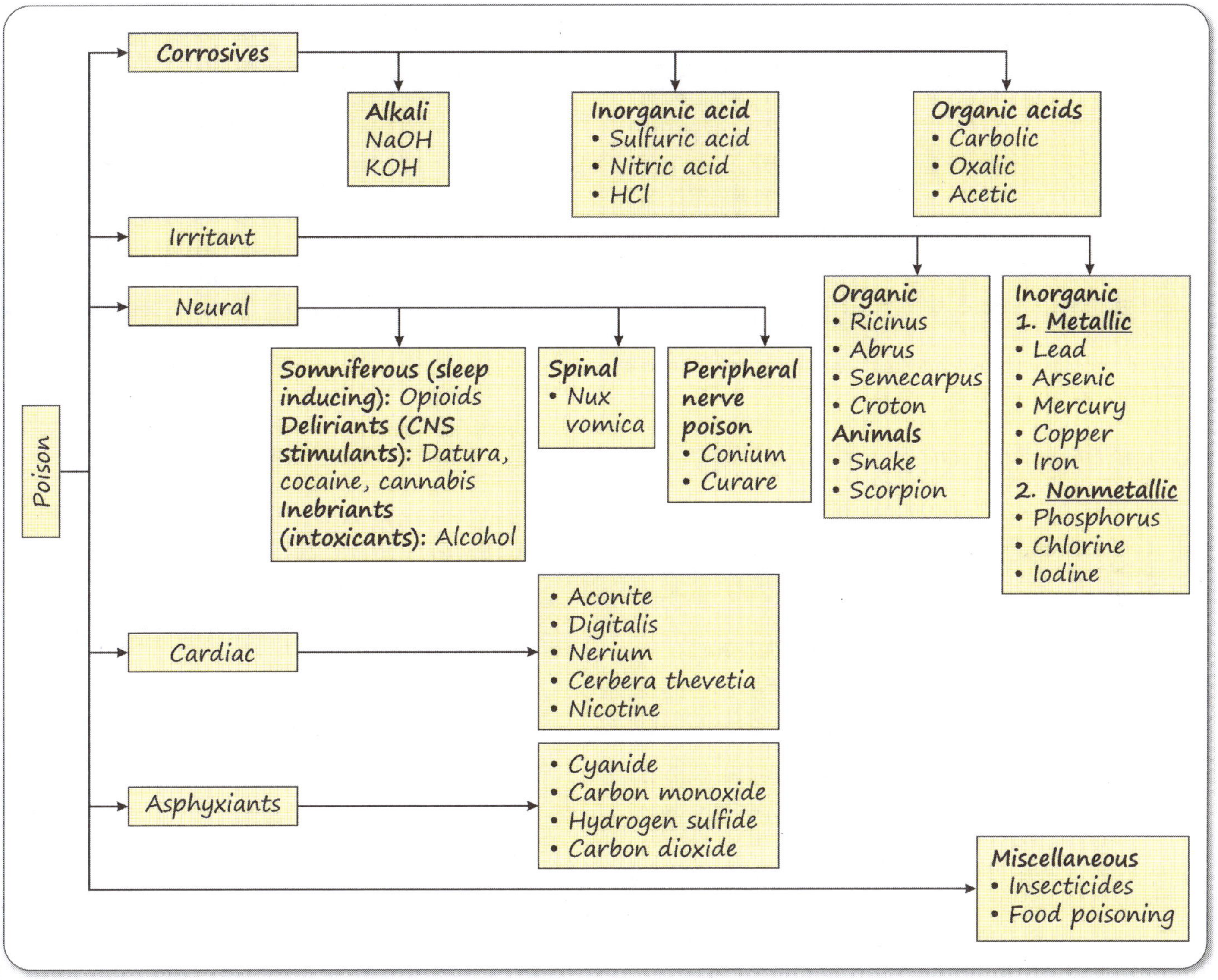

Poisoning from Postmortem Findings

Hypostasis color	Smell	Teeth and gums	Stomach mucosa
• Carbon monoxide: Cherry red • Cyanide: Brick red • Phosphorus: Dark brown • Bromide, aniline and nitrites: Chocolate brown • Aniline: Deep blue • Hydroen sulfide: Bluish green • Opium: Black • Methanol: Purple	• Cyanide: Oil of bitter almonds • Cannabis: Burnt rope • Hydroen sulfide: Rotten egg • Alcohol: Fruity odor • Chloralhydrate and paraldehyde: Acrid pear • Organophosphates: Kerosene/garlic odor • Phosphorus, arsenic: Garlic odor • Conium maculatum (Hemlock): Mousy • Salicylates: Oil of winter green	• Chalky white teeth: Sulfuric acid • Yellow teeth: Nitric acid • Bluish deposits in gums: Lead, mercury, iron, sliver • Green deposits in gums: Copper	• Sulfuric acid: Black necrotic mucosa • Sulfuric acid: Wet blotting paper stomach. • Nitric acid: Yellow or brown • Carbolic acid (phenol): Hardened Leathery mucosa. • Arsenic: Red velvety mucosa. • Mercury: Slate gray mucosa • Copper sulphate and sodium amytal: Bluish mucosa

Viscera preservation/chemical analysis of viscera (Please refer thanatology chapter).

DUTIES OF A DOCTOR

- **Medical duties:** To treat the patient.
- **Legal duties:** To follow the legal formalities.

Legal Duties

Legal duties of a doctor include the following:

- Collect and preserve evidences (Ex: Food samples, stained clothing, stained vomitus, gastric lavage fluid)
    - Intentionally not preserving evidence (causing disappearance of evidence)—Punishable under 201 IPC.
- If the patient is serious, arrange for dying declaration.
- Do not issue death certificate, in case of death.
- Intimation to police:
    - Suspicious cases, homicidal cases, accidental cases and suicide cases with suspected foul play must be informed to the police as per 39 CrPC.
    - Failure to inform by doctor → Punishable under 176 IPC
    - Falsely informing police → Punishable under 177 IPC
- Attempt to commit suicide is not a crime.

GENERAL GUIDELINES IN THE MEDICAL MANAGEMENT OF A CASE OF POISONING

- **Stabilization:** Airway, breathing, circulation.
- Removal of unabsorbed poisons (decontaminatin).
- Neutralisation with antidotes.
- Symptomatic measures.

Decontamination: Depending on the route of exposure

- **Skin contact:** Wash with water.
- **Inhalational:** Move the patient to fresh air.
- **Oral route:** Emesis, gastric lavage, catharsis, activated charcoal, whole bowel irrigation.

Gastric Lavage

- Very effective within 1 hour of poison ingestion.
- **Position:** Left lateral position or sitting position.
- **Tubes:** Lavacuator (best), Ewald's tube, Boas tube, Ryles tube.

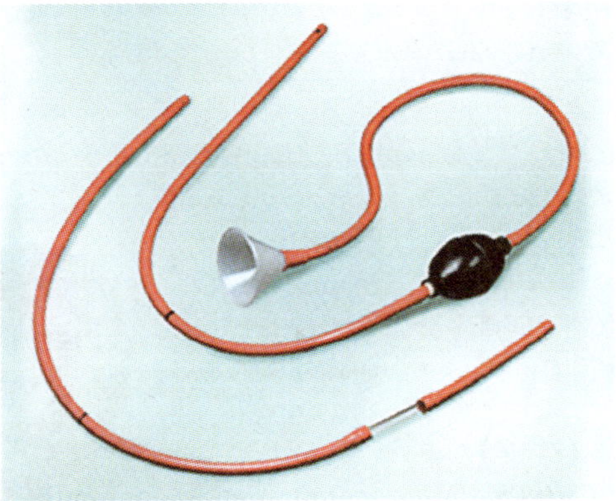

Contraindications

- Corrosives (except carbolic acid)
- Comatose patients
- Convulsant poisons (strychnos nux vomica)
- Esophageal varices
- Volatile poisons (kerosene/petroleum distillates)

Activated Charcoal (Mechanical Antidote)

- Contains small pores with larger surface areas.
- The pores **adsorb**[Q] the poisons
- 1 g of activated carbon has surface area of 3,000 m^2

Enhanced Elimination of Absorbed Poison

- Multi dose activated charcoal
  - Repeated administration of charcoal to enhance elimination of toxins/drugs that have already been absorbed into the body and drugs with enterohepatic circulation.
  - Useful for drugs like carbamazepine, digitalis, phenobarbital etc.
- Hemodialysis
- Urinary alkalinization: Preferred for excretion of acidic drugs: (salicylates[Q], phenobarbitone)
- Urinary acidification: Preferred for alkaloid drugs (not routinely used).

ANTIDOTES

• Acetaminophen: N-acetyl cysteine • Datura: Physostigmine • Arsenic: BAL (dimercaprol) • DMSA (succimer) • β-blocker: Glucagon • Benzodiazepine: Flumazenil • Copper: D-penicillamine • Cocaine: Amylnitrite • Carbon monoxide: High flow oxygen, hyperbaric oxygen	• Cyanide: Nitrites (amylnitrite and sodium nitrite) • Hydroxycobalamin • Digitalis, oleander: Digibind • Heparin: Protamine sulphate • Iron: Desferrioaxamine, Defeperidone • Lead: EDTA ▪ (Severe Poisoning: EDTA + BAL/ DMSA) • Morphine: Nalaxone • Methanol: Fomepizole/Ethanol	• Oxalic acid: Calcium gluconate • OPC: Atropine and Oximes • Carbamates: Atropine • Snake bite: Neostigmine • Scorpion sting: prazosin • Spider bite: prazosin

CORROSIVES (CAUSTICS)

Corrosives Tissue Damage

- Voluntarily causing grievous hurt by acids—**Sec. 326A IPC**[Q] (10 years/life imprisonment)
- Attempt of vitriolage—**Sec. 326 B IPC**[Q] (5-7 years)

Acids	
Inorganic acid Only local effects	**Organic acid** Local and systemic effects
• Sulfuric acid • Nitric acid • Hydrochloric acid	• Carbolic acid • Oxalic acid • Acetic acid

Alkalis
Ammonia **Carbonates** of sodium and potassium **Hydroxides** of sodium and potassium

Vitriolage: Throwing of any corrosive with intention to disfigure

Burns
- Chemical burns on face
- Painless
- Skin corroded and ulcerated
- No singeing of hair
- Vesicles (rare)
- Contractures common

Topical management
- Irrigation with NS or water
- Topical MgO
- **Eye:** Olive oil
- Symptomatic measures

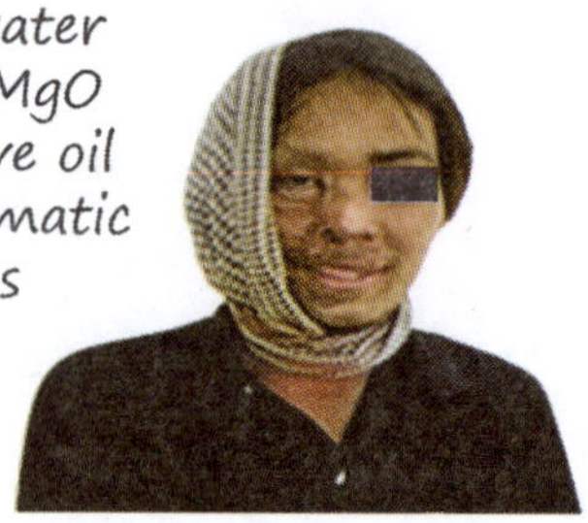

Sulfuric acid (oil of vitrial/battery acids)	**Nitric acid** (aqua fortis)
Hygroscopic property **Only local effects** **PM Findings** • Black charred tongue • Chalky white teeth[Q] • Black charred stomach mucosa • Wet blotting paper stomach[Q] • Stomach perforation common	**Xanthoproteic reacion:** Picric acid formation (yellow color) **PM Findings** • Yellow skin staining/yellow teeth • Yellow/brown stomach mucosa

Phenol (carbolic acid)
- Antiseptic/disinfectant
- Phenolic/hospital odor

Acute poisoning: Carbolism **Chronic poisoning:** Phenolic marasmus

Deposition in ligaments/skin/cornea resulting in black pigmentation: **Ochronosis**

↑ Metabolites

Phenol → **Stomach** → **Pyrocatechol hydroquinone** →

*Absorption via all routes

Buff white/ leathery mucosa

C – CNS depression
C – Convulsions
C – Constricted pupil
C – CV shock

C – Convoluted tubule damage
C – Carboluria[Q] (olive green color urine[Q])

Management:
- Decontamination
- Management of convulsions/shock/ arrhythmia

***Phenol delays putrefaction**

Oxalic acid (carbolic acid)	• Used in ink remover[Q] solution (used to erase writing in attempts at forgery[Q]) • Present in vegetables like spinach and cabbage

Local effects

Oxalic acid → Stomach

- Burning pain
- Coffee ground vomitus

→ *Absorption in blood →

Systemic effects

*Oxalic acid combines with calcium to form calcium oxalates

- Oxaluria (excretion of casts in urine)
  Postal envelope shape casts
- Tubular precipitation of casts
  ↓
  PCT damage
  ↓
  Renal failure

- Hypocalcemia
- Tetany

Management:
- Gastric lavage with calcium lactate
- Antidote: Calcium gluconate (IV)

Hydrofluoric Acid

Produces fluoride ions and hydrogen ions	Mechanism	Effects
	Liquefactive necrosis	Severe local pain Deep dermal burns
	Combines with calcium and magnesium to form insoluble salts	Hypocalcemia Hypomagnesemia Hyperkalemia

METALS IRRITANTS

Arsenic (Metalloid)

Toxic Compounds of Arsenic from Highest to Lowest Toxicity

- Arsine gas (most toxic form)
- Inorganic arsenic (e.g., arsenic trioxide—most toxic salt, inheritance powder)
- Organic arsenic
- Elemental arsenic

Types of poisoning

Fulminant (massive dose 3 g)	Acute (large doses)	Chronic (small doses over long time)
Sudden death due to cardiovascular collapse	**Gastroenteritis type and narcotic type** • Presenting with abdominal pain and severe loose stools • Symptoms resemble cholera • CNS features **Autopsy findings** **Stomach:** • Hemorrhagic gastritis • Red velvety stomach mucosa	**Arsenicosis** **Hydroarsenicsm** (due to drinking arsenic-contaminated water) • Occupational—miners/smelters • Homicidal—food/drink

Clinical Features

A – Alopecia

Aldrich Mees line[Q]: White bands of opacity in the nails of fingers and toes

R – Rain drop pigmentation[Q] – Brown pigmentation over skin flexures, temples, shoulders, palm, eyelids and neck

S – Skin Rash (resembling measles)

E (skin) Eruptions – Hyperkeratosis[Q] of the palms and soles bilaterally.

N – Neuropathy (sensorimotor neuropathy) – Peripheral neuropathy with tingling, numbness of hands and feet (glove and stocking distribution[Q])

Nasal Septal Perforation

I – Ischemia in peripheries due to vasospasm –

- Chronic exposure also causes vasospasm and peripheral vascular insufficiency
- Dry gangrene and spontaneous amputations of affected extremities—(BLACK FOOT DISEASE[Q])

C – Carcinogenic (BCC, SCC, lung, liver and bladder)

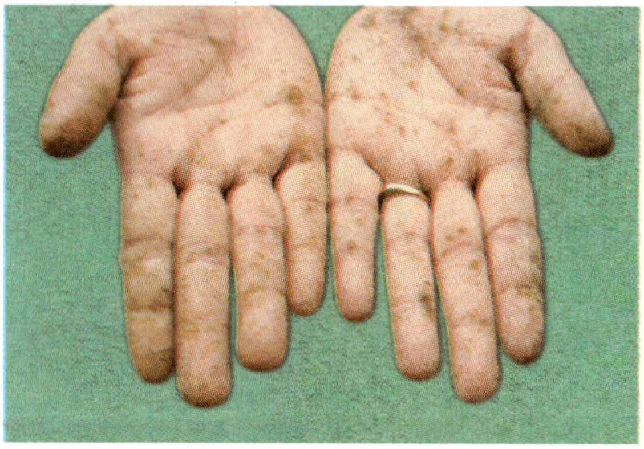

Diagnosis of Arsenic Toxicity

- Acute poisoning: **Blood sample**[Q] **and urine sample (more reliable)**
- Chronic poisoning: **Hair, nail and bone**[Q]
- Marsh test[Q], Reinsch[Q] test
- **Recent:** Atomic absorption spectroscopy and neutron activation analysis

Disadvantages of Arsenic Usage as Homicidal Poison

- It delays putrefaction[Q].
- Can be detected in completely decomposed bodies[Q].
- Can be found in bones[Q], hairs[Q] and nails for several years.
- Can be detected in charred bones or ashes[Q].

Mercury (Quick Silver)

Predisposed Occupation: Workers of hat industries[Q] (Hatter's shakes[Q]) and glass blowing industries (Glass Blower's shakes)

Chronic mercury poisoning is **Hydragyrism**[Q].

[**Toxicity:** Organic mercury > Mercuric salts[Q] > Mercurous salts]

Mnemonic:

Hg METAL

H – Hatters

G – Glass blowers/gingivitis

M – Minamata disease

E – Erethism +

T – Tremors

Acrodynia

L – Lentis (mercuria lentis)

Features of Chronic Mercury Poisoning

Elemental mercury	Organic mercury (most toxic form)	Inorganic	
Not toxic orally (not absorbed in GIT) Inhalational (vapor form): Toxic Acute exposure to fumes: METAL FUME FEVER (illness similar to Kawasaki disease)	**Methyl mercury** • Minamata disease • (Also causes Hunter-Russel syndrome)	**Mercuric salts (more toxic salt)** • Mercuric chloride • Mercuric sulfide • Mercuric thiocyanate	**Mercuric salts (less toxic salt)** • Mercuric chloride • Mercuric sulfide • Mercuric thiocyanate

MINAMATA DISEASE (by Methyl mercury)

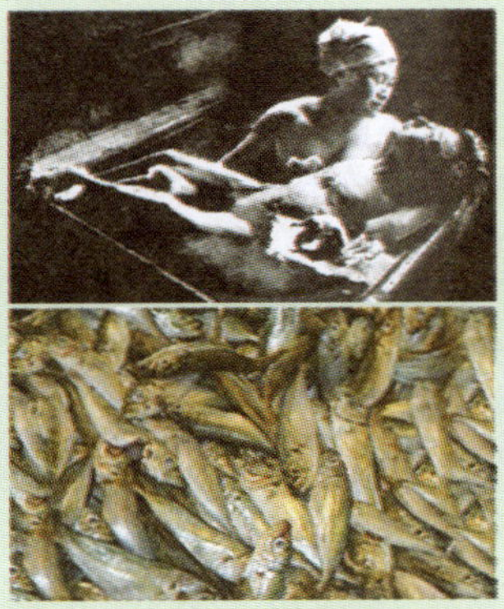

- Chronic organic mercury intoxication caused by eating contaminated fish and shellfish[Q]
- Symptoms include disturbances in hand coordination, gait and speech.

Extra Edge

Tremors

Coarse intentional tremors[Q] (**Danbury tremors/ Hatter's shakes/Glass Blower's shakes**[Q])

Site: First in the **hands**[Q] → lips → tongue →arms and legs.

Features

- Worsening of handwriting—early feature
- In the advanced stage, the person is unable to dress himself, write legibly or walk properly.
- Most severe form of tremors is **concussion mercurialis**

Mecurialentis

Mechanism: Brownish deposition of mercury in anterior lens capsule[Q]

Site: Anterior lens capsule, bilateral

Slit lamp examination: Malt brown reflex[Q].

Visual acuity: Normal (**no effect on visual acuity**[Q])

ERETHISM

- Mad Hatter syndrome
- Neuropsychiatric symptoms[Q]
- Personality change, irritability, shyness, dementia, insomnia

Acrodynia (Pink Disease)/Swift-Feer Disease/ Calomel Disease

Toxicity:

- Idiosyncratic hypersensitivity[Q] reaction to mercurous chloride[Q] (calomel)

Age group: Children[Q]

Contd...

Features

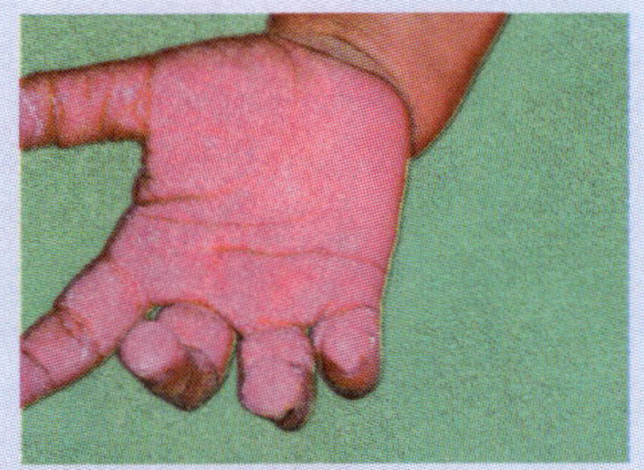

- Pink discoloration in the hands and feet
  - Pink
  - Puffy
  - Painful
  - Paraesthetic peripheries
- Associated with dental fillings, teething powders

Lead (Shisha)

Toxic Forms

Organic (most toxic form): lead tetroxide	Inorganic form
Antiknock in petrol Lead encephalopathy[Q]	Lead acetate—Most common source of lead poisoning[Q] Lead sulfide—**Least toxic form**[Q] Lead carbonate—Paints **Lead tetroxide (most toxic salt)**—Used as Sindoor

Plumbism/Saturnism—*Chronic Lead Poisoning*

Most common chronic heavy metal poisoning.

Most common route: Adult—Inhalational[Q] in occupational exposure and children: Oral

Mnemonic:

Plumbism Features

ABCDEFG

A – Anemia

B – Burtonian line/basophilic stippling, bone lines (**lead lines**)

C – Colic, constipation (dry belly ache), Cabot's ring

D – Drop (wrist/foot drop)—**Lead palsy** (nerve degeneration)

E – Encephalopathy

F – Facial pallor (earliest sign)

G – Gout (**saturnine gout**)

Anemia
Microcytic hypochromic anemia
Inhibition of ALA dehydrataseQ and ferrochelatase

Burtonian line
- Blue line along gumsQ
- Opposite to caries toothQ
- Deposition of lead sulfideQ (lead + H_2S by bacteria)

Punctate basophilia/ basophilic stippling
Lead inhibits Pyrimidine 5 nucleotidase → RibosomesQ aggregates as dark blue spots in RBC cytoplasmQ

Bone line/lead line/ lead osteopathy
- Among childrenQ
- **Deposition of calcium in growing ends of bonesQ**
- **RadiopaqueQ bands** along metaphysisQ of long bones

Colic (saturnine colic, painter's colic)
NocturnalQ
SpasmodicQ abdominal pain lasting for a few minutes

Lead encephalopathy
Due to **tetra ethyl lead**
- **In childrenQ**
- Irritability, restlessness, hallucinations and coma
- **Brain damage is irreversible and permanentQ**

Ouch DiseaseQ
(**Ita Ita disease** = "it hurts-it hurts disease")
- Due to cadmium toxicity.
- Weak and brittle bones.
- Spinal and leg pain is common
- Osteomalacia—Bones weaken resulting in multiple pathological bone fractures

NONMETALLIC IRRITANTS

Phosphorus

White phosphorus (yellow phosphorus)	Red phosphorus
Toxic	Non toxic
luminousQ in dark (phosphorescence)	Nonluminous
Garlic odor	Odorless
Inflammable (unstable, should be kept under water)	Noninflammable
Emits smoke	No smoke

Acute phosphorus poisoning	Chronic phosphorus poisoning
• **Garlicky odorQ**. • **Luminous vomit and stoolQ** because of the presence of phosphorus. • Fumes emanate from the stools (**smoking or smoky stool syndromeQ**). • Acute poisoning causes liver cell necrosis, **fatty liverQ** and acute yellow atrophy.	**Phossy Jaw/Glass Jaw/Lucifer's Jaw** Due to **inhalation of fumes** over years. **Tooth ache (earliest symptomQ)** → swelling of the jaw → OsteoNecrosis **of lower jawQ** → multiple sinuses discharging foul-smelling pus. 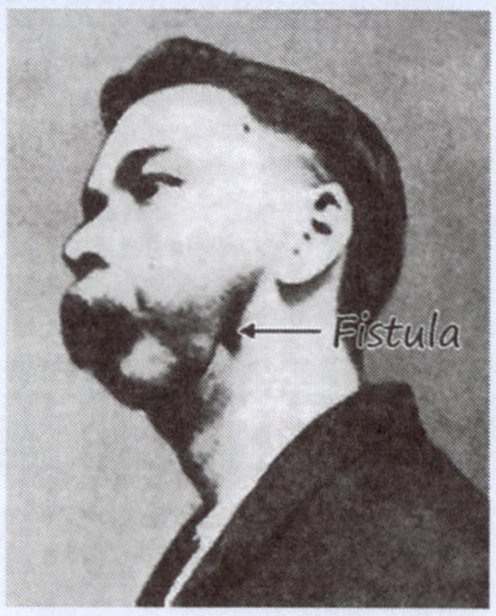

ORGANIC IRRITANTS

Plant Irritants

- **Plant irritants do not have antidotes[Q], except Abrin (antiabrin[Q]—antidote)**
- **Symptomatic management only**

	Ricinus communis (castor)	Abrus precatorius (Gunchi/ Rati/rosary bead/Indian Liquorice)	Croton tiglium	Semecarpus anacardium/ Bhilawa (Marking Nut)	Calotropis gigantea	Capsicum annum/ chilli
	• Unbroken seeds are not poisonous. • Crushing of seeds yields Castor oil (nontoxic) and residue (toxic)	Seeds are bright scarlet red with a black spot at one pole	• Seeds resemble castor. • Croton seeds when crushed yield oil (toxic) and residue (toxic).	Seeds are black heart-shaped with a rough projection at the base.		
Active Principle:	**Ricin[Q]**	**Abrin[Q]** Others: Abrine, abric acid and abraline	• **Crotin[Q]** • **Crotonic acid** • **Crotonoside**	**Semicarpol and Bhilawanol[Q]**	Calactin, calotoxin and calotropin[Q]	• Capsicin • Capsaicin
	Ricin is a biological warfare agent (category B[Q]) 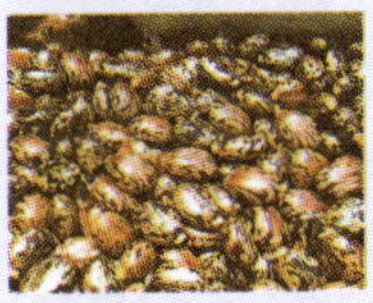	• Similar to **Viper snake venom[Q]** • Used as **SUI needles[Q]** • **Anti abrin[Q]** (antidote) • Ideal cattle poison 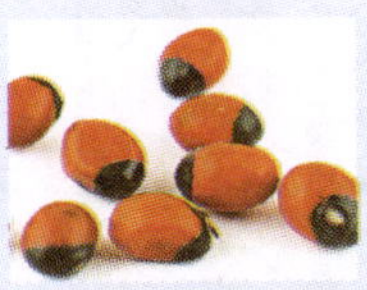	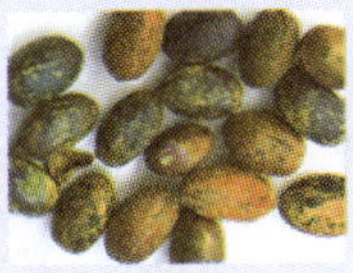	To produce **artificial bruise/ conjunctivitis[Q]** **Applied to the skin:** Irritation, itching and a painful blister[Q] with acrid serum[Q]. The lesion resembles a bruise. 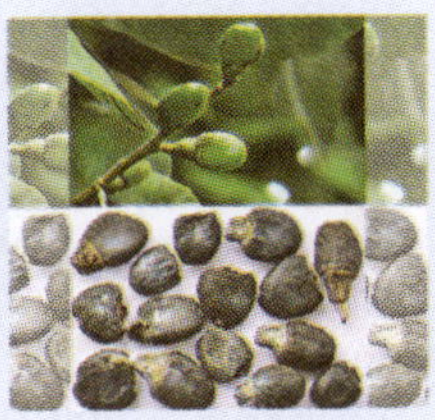	Skin: Blister Eye: Conjunctivitis and blindness Ingestion: Vomiting and diarrhea Calotropis root—highly poisonous to cobras and other poisonous snakes. 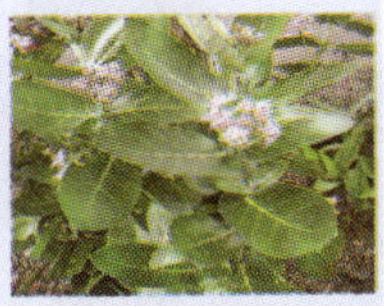	Used for torture/ robbery. **Hunan's hand syndrome**—painful Contact dermatitis to chilli powder exposure. 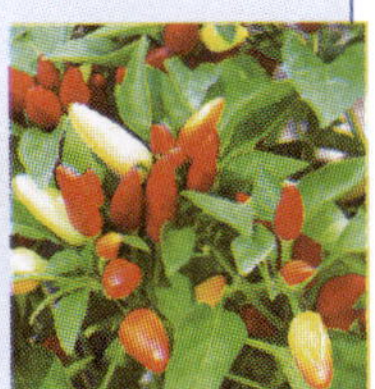

Sui Needles

- Powdered **abrus seeds** mixed with dhatura and opium and made into paste with spirit and water.

- Sharp needles are made from this paste and dried under sun.
- The cattle are struck with needles (so as to **resemble snakebite**).
- Painful swelling develops at the site of injection, with inflammation and necrosis, sepsis and death.
- The sui needle injection resembles **viperine snake bite**[Q].

ANIMAL IRRITANT: SNAKES

Appearance	Venomous snakes	Nonvenomous snakes (mostly)
Habit	**Nocturnal**	**Not specific**
Head scales	Usually small[Q] Three exceptions (poisonous snakes with large head scales) • Cobra • Krait **Cobra:** 3rd supra labial touches eye and nasal shields **Krait:** Four infralabials scales below mouth and 4th being largest	Usually large
Belly scales	Large and cover the entire breadth of belly[Q]	Small
Tail	Compressed[Q]	Not compressed
Fangs	Long and canalized, like hypodermic needle	Short or small grooved teeth
Bite mark	Two fang marks[Q]	Small teeth marks[Q]

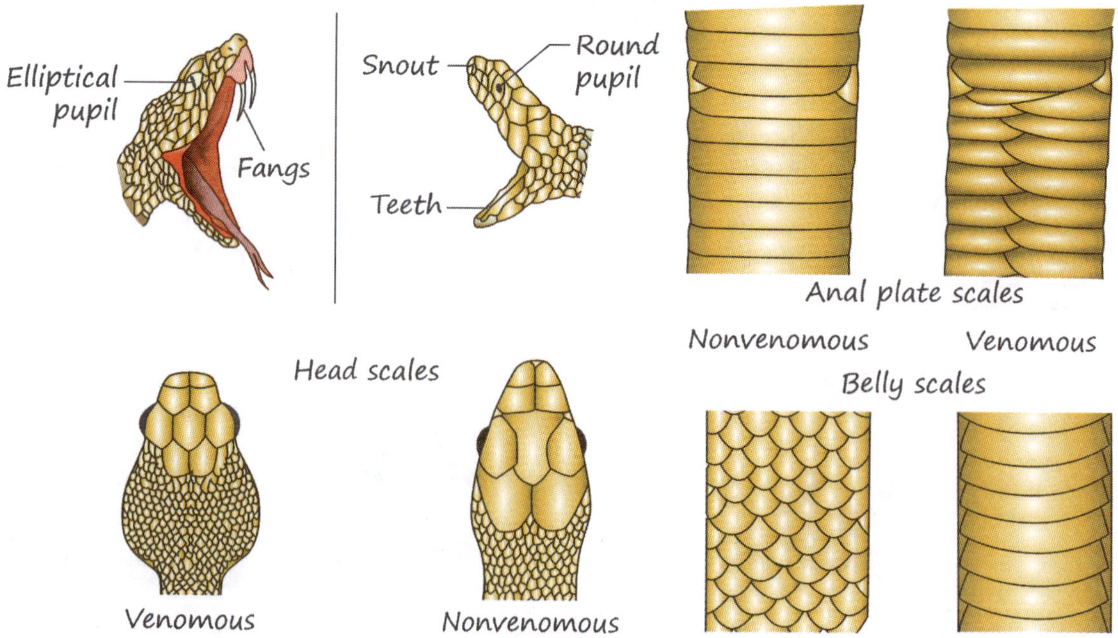

Venomous snakes

- **Elapidae (neurotoxic)**
  - King cobra (Ophiophagus hannah)
  - Common cobra (Naja naja)
  - Common krait (Bungarus caeruleus)
- **Viperidae (hemotoxic)**
  - Russell's viper (Daboia russeli)
  - Saw scaled viper (Echnis carinate)
- **Hydrophidae (myotoxic)**
  - Sea snake

Ophiology[Q]: Study of snakes; **Ophitoxaemia**[Q]: Circulation of snake venom in blood.

Four venomous snake species are responsible for most of the human snake bite cases in the India.

The big four

1. **Indian cobra, Naja naja**[Q]
2. **Common krait, Bungarus caeruleus**[Q]
3. **Russell's viper, Daboia russelii**[Q]
4. **Saw-scaled viper, Echis carinatus**[Q]

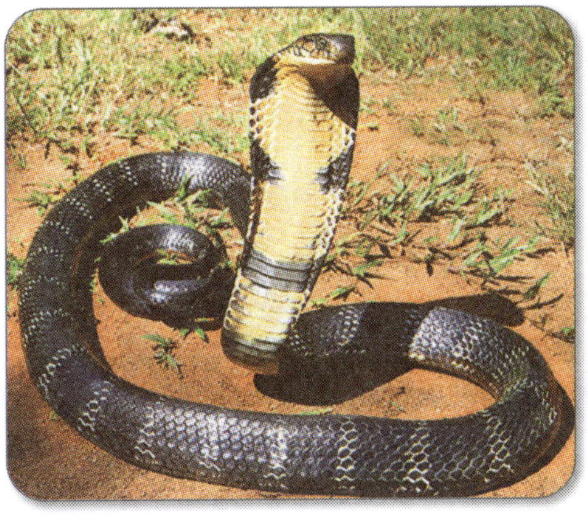

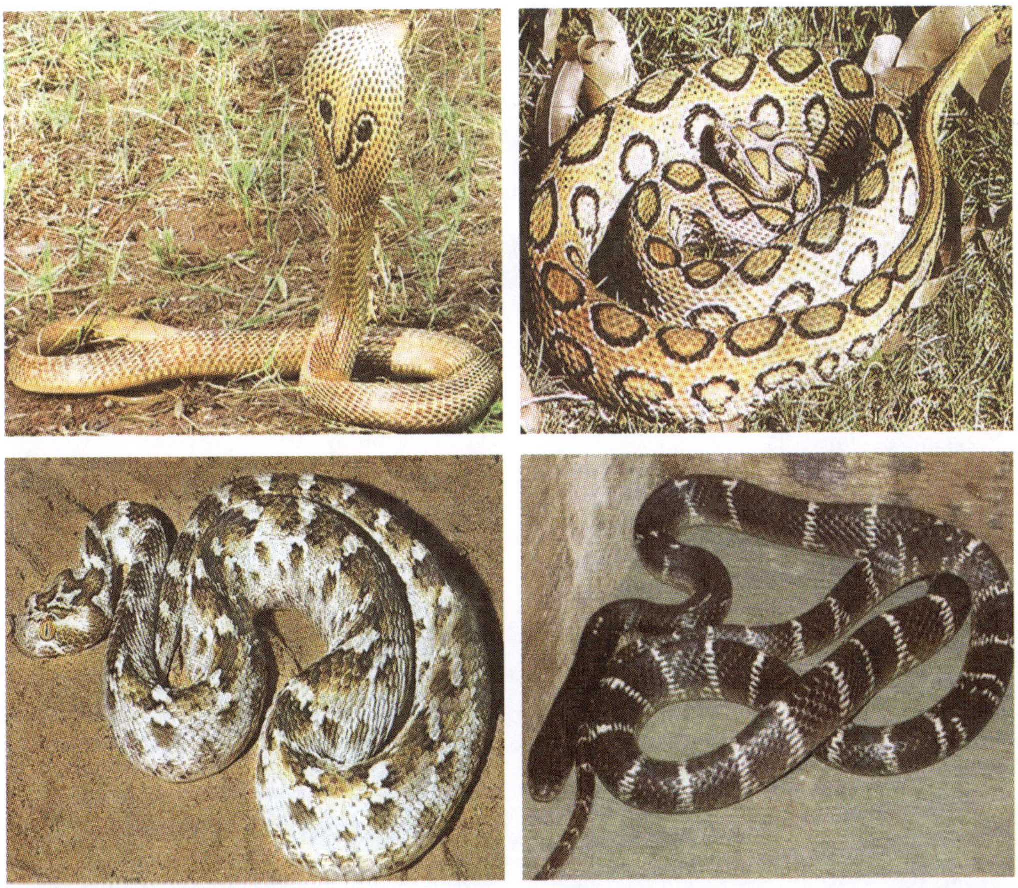

Clinical Features

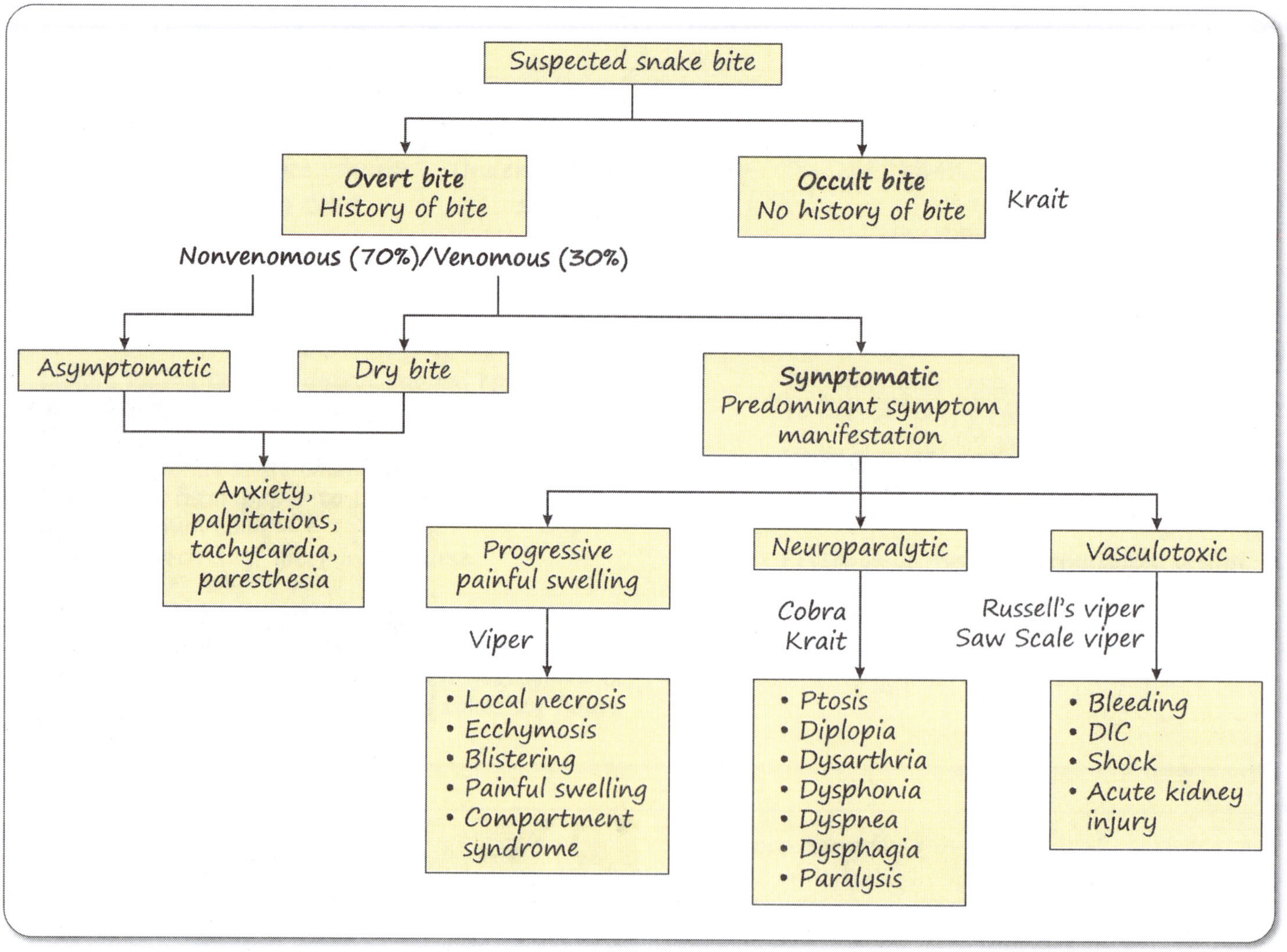

Management of Snake Bite

First aid approach	Specific Rx
"CARRY NO RIGHT" No → No incision/suction No tourniquet/ligature No electrotherapy No coffee/alcohol Right → R → Reassurance I → Immobilization (pressure) (Sutherland's Wrap) G → get to hospital H → T → Tell the doctor of systemic toxic signs	1. ASV (antisnake venom) Source: Horse serum (it gives allergic symptoms) Test dose Not needed Effective against: Big 4 snakes **Indian Antisnake venom is effective against** ▪ Cobra[Q] ▪ Krait[Q] ▪ Russell's viper[Q] ▪ Saw scaled viper[Q] Route → IV Dose → 10 vials 2. IV neostigmine ▪ It will reverse the neuroparalysis ↓ Only for cobra bite

Extra Edge

20-Minute Whole Blood Clotting Test (20 WBCT)

- The **most reliable**[Q] **test** of venom-induced defibrinogenation.
- A few milliliters of venous blood is put in a clean test tube and kept aside for 20 minutes.
- It is then tilted to see if it has clotted or not.
- Incoagulability indicates systemic envenomation by vipers.

INEBRIANTS

Alcohol

Toxicity: Isopropyl alcohol > Methyl alcohol[Q] **> Ethyl alcohol**

Ethanol

Ratio of blood alcohol with different body fluids	Methods to find blood and urine alcohol levels
• Blood: Urine = 1:1.33 • Blood: Exhaled air (breath) = 1:2300 • Blood: Saliva = 1:12 • Blood: CSF = 1:1.17	• **Kozelka and Hine test**[Q] • **Cavett test**[Q] • **Gas chromatography (most specific**[Q]**)** • **Statutory limit for driving in India: 30 mg%**[Q] (Sec. 185 of Motor Vehicles Act) • **Public nuisance** under the influence of alcohol is punishable under **Sec. 510 IPC** • Abrupt excess or stoppage of alcohol can cause **delirium tremens (Mania a Potu)** • **Any crime committed by a person suffering from delirium tremens, is not punishable.**

Methanol (Wood Alcohol)—Responsible for HOOCH tragedy

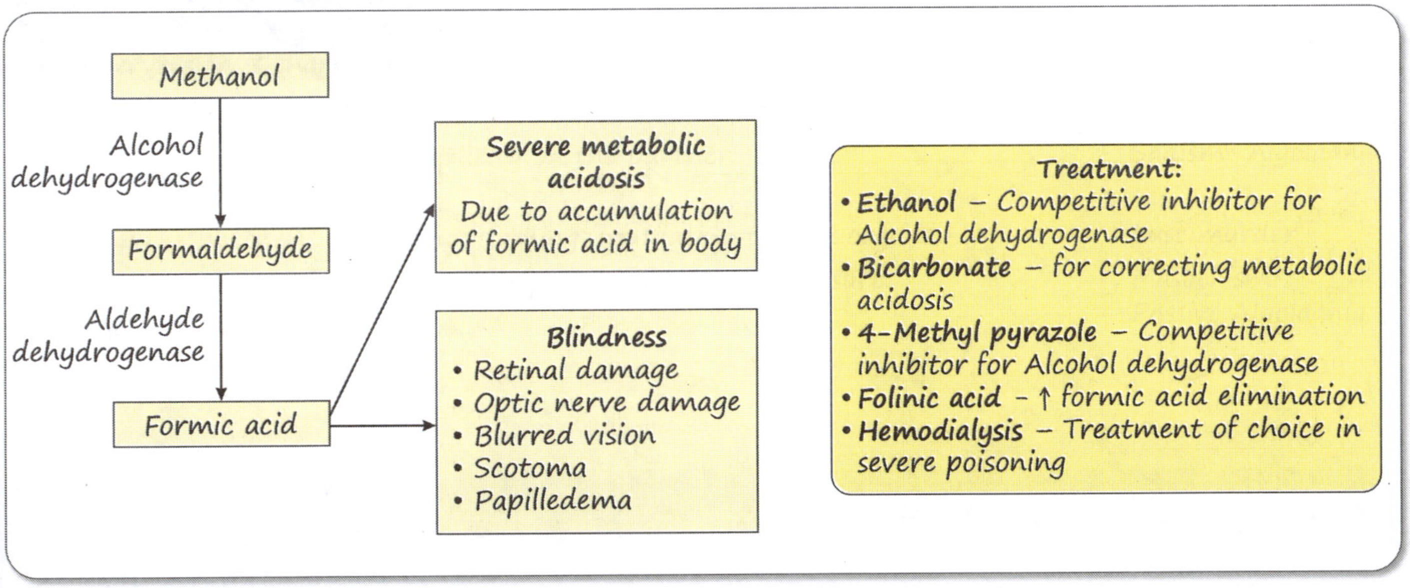

Opium/Afim/Madak/Chandu

- Opium (poppy) is derived from Papaver somniferum.
- The juice is obtained by cutting the unripe capsule. It is dried to a brown residue (**crude residue**).
- Poppy seeds are used for cooking and are nontoxic
- Triad of morphine poisoning: Coma + Pinpoint pupil + Respiratory depression
- Antidote: Nalaxone sodium

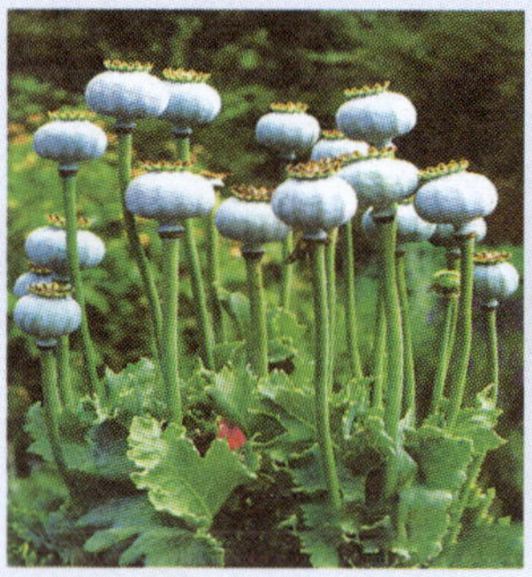

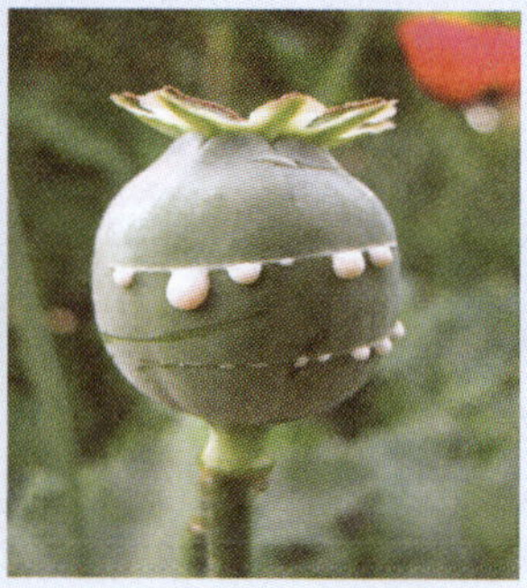

Heroin/Smack/Junk/Dope/Brown Sugar

Brown Sugar/Junk/Smack/Dope

Semisynthetic derivative of morphine

Diacetyl morphine

Methods of Abuse

- IV injection: Mainlining
- Skin injection: skin popping
- Inhaling the vapor: chasing the dragon

Speed ball → Heroine + Cocaine

Hot shot → Heroine + Strychnine

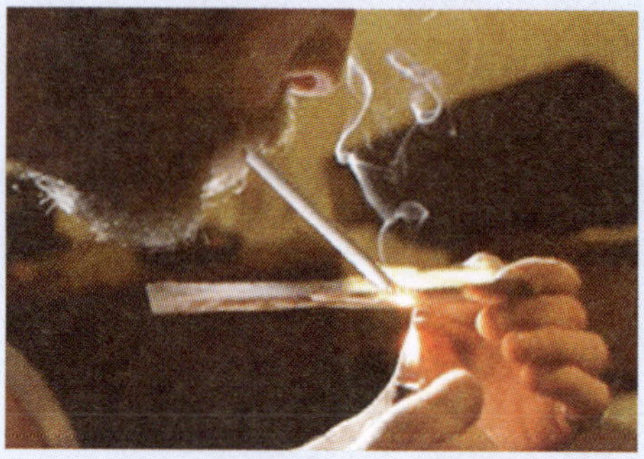

DELIRIANTS

Datura: Three varieties: Datura alba (white flowers); Datura Niger (purple flower); Datura stramonium

All parts are toxic. Roots and seeds most toxic.

Datura fruit is thorn apple[Q].

Active principle: Atropine[Q], Hyoscyamine[Q] and Scopolamine[Q]

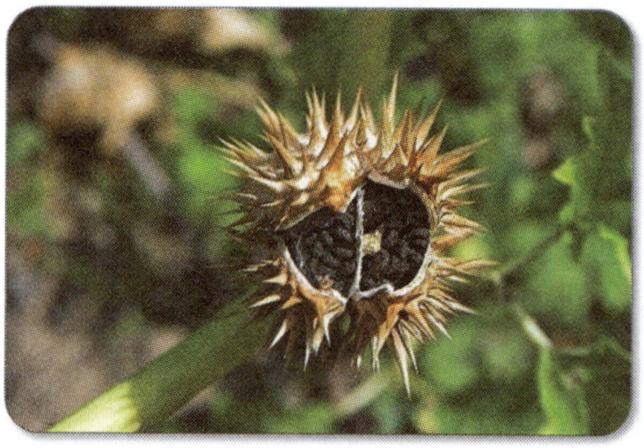

Mnemonic: **Datura Poisoning**

9'Ds

1. Dilated pupils
2. Dry skin
3. Dry mouth
4. Dysphagia
5. Dysphasia
6. Drunken gait
7. Drowsiness
8. Delirium
9. Death

Carphologia[Q] present

Treatment: Physostigmine is the antidote of choice

- Stupefying agent: used by criminals to the passengers prior to robbery, rape or kidnapping.
- Road side poison and Railway poison:
- Accidental Poisoning: As datura seeds resemble chilly seeds.

Cannabis (Indian Hemp)

Street names: Pot, Weed, Rope, Dope, Joint, Hash, Reefer.

Active Principle: Cannabidiol which is inert, is converted to active **tetrahydrocannabinols**[Q] (THC) on exposure to heat

Preparations	Source	Active principal percentage	
Bhang	Dried leaves and stem	<15%	**Majoon** • Sweet prepared from bhang
Ganja	Dried flowers	15–25%	Smoked in the form of cigarette: **Joint/Reefer**
Hashis/Charas	Dried resin	25–40%	
Hash oil	Resin	60–70%	Most potent form of cannabis

Chronic Cannabis Poisoning: Mnemonic: FAVORITE

F – Flashback phenomenon (sudden recurrence of effects of cannabis (even if when not used)

A – **Amotivational syndrome**

VO – Vomiting (Hyperemesis syndrome – Excessive nausea and vomiting)

R – Run amok

Homicidal impulse to kill[Q]

Act: The addict first kills a person against whom he may have real enmity and then kills anyone who comes in his way, until the homicidal tendency lasts.

Criminal Responsibility

The person is **not held responsible**[Q] for his acts since 'run amok' is considered a disorder of mind and not intoxication.

I – Insanity (**hashish insanity/Hemp insanity**)

TE – Testosterone decrease resulting in loss of libido.

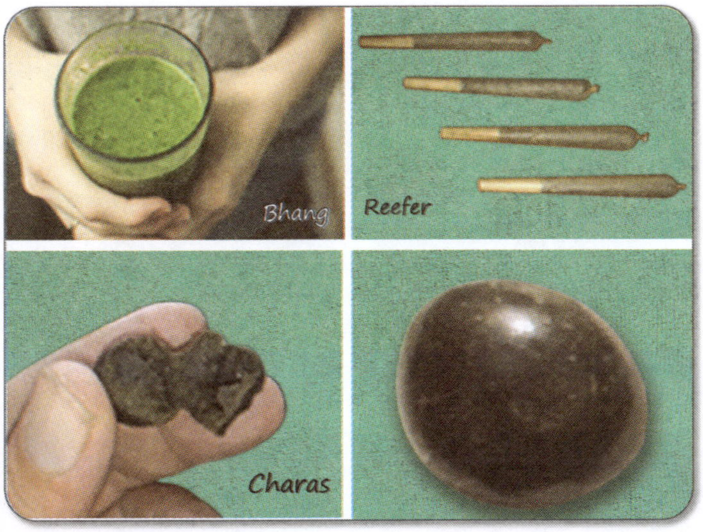

Cocaine Poisoning

('Coke', 'Snow', 'Cadillac', 'White lady')

- Alkaloid deliriant, obtained from dried leaves of Erythroxylum coca

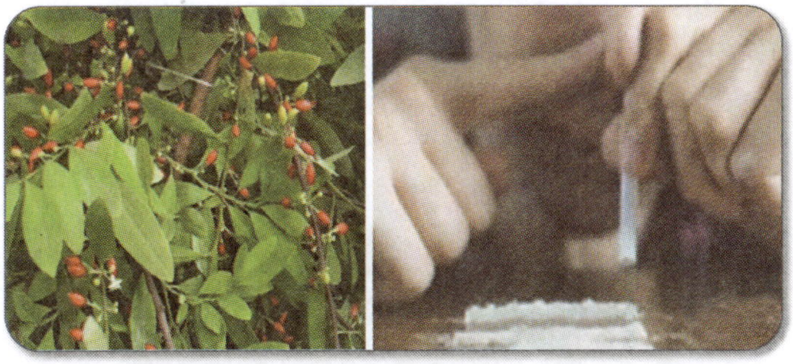

Actions of Cocaine

Cocaine induces hyperadrenergic[Q] state

Local anesthetic[Q]

Intense vasoconstrictor[Q] leads to stroke, cardiac infarction and ischemic colitis.

Dilated pupils, hyperthermia

Body Packer Syndrome/Mini Packer Syndrome

- **Body packer/Mule:** An individual who ingests and smuggles packets of illicit drugs such as **cocaine**[Q] to transport them.
- During the transport, rupture of the packet releases cocaine into GIT and absorbed into circulation suddenly and causing acute cocaine poisoning.
- Person may die of myocardial infarction or intracerebral hemorrhage

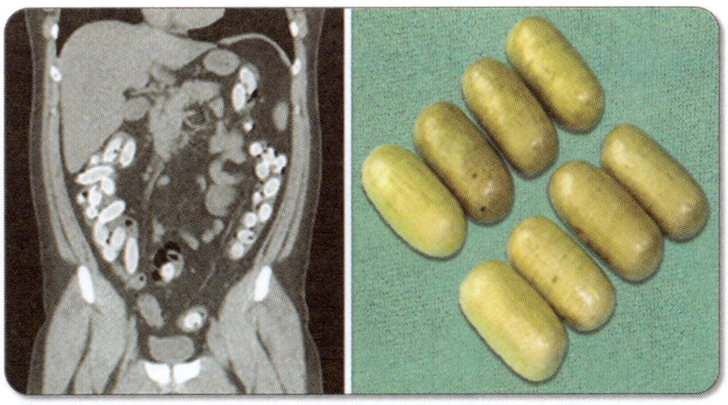

Chronic Cocaine Abuse (Cocainism/Cocainophagia/Cocainomania)

Black tongue[Q] **and Teeth**
Nasal septal perforation[Q] (due to chronic snorting)
Palatal perforation[Q] (due to placing cocaine under the palate)
Gangrene[Q] in peripheries (ear pinna, nose tip, etc.)

Magnan's Syndrome/Cocaine Bugs
- Tactile hallucination[Q].
- Feeling of Small insects are creeping on the skin
- Giving rise to itching sensation (**formication**).

SPINAL POISON- STRYCHNOS NUX-VOMICA

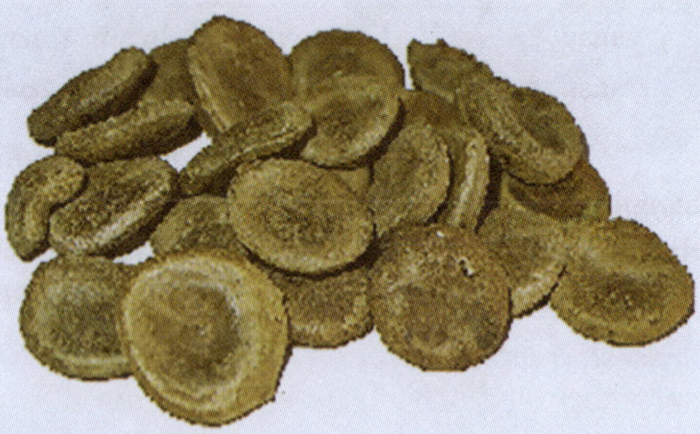

Kuchila Seeds/Dogs buttons:
- Seeds are flat, **circular disks**[Q], concave on one side and convex on the other, covered with silky hairs.
- They resemble enlarged RBCs.
- Intact seeds are not toxic, only crushed seeds are toxic.
- 1 crushed seed can be fatal.

Active Principles

- **Strychnine**[Q]—Alkaloid
- **Brucine**[Q]—Alkaloid
- Loganin—Glucoside

Toxic Action

Strychnine competitively **antagonizes glycine**[Q] (inhibitory neurotransmitter) in the **anterior horn**[Q] **cells of spinal cord (Renshaw cells**).

Clinical Features

- **Increased rigidity of muscles** and muscular twitching.
- **Convulsions:** Initially, clonic but eventually become tonic, and affect all the muscles at the same time.
- In between convulsions, **muscles are completely relaxed**[Q] and breathing is resumed.
- **Consciousness is not lost**[Q] and the mind remains clear till death.

- ***Risus Sardonicus***[Q]
- ***Opisthotonus***[Q]*: Backward bending of the body*
- ***Emprosthotonus***[Q]*: Forward bending of the body.*
- ***Pleurosthotonus***[Q]*: Sideward bending of the body.*

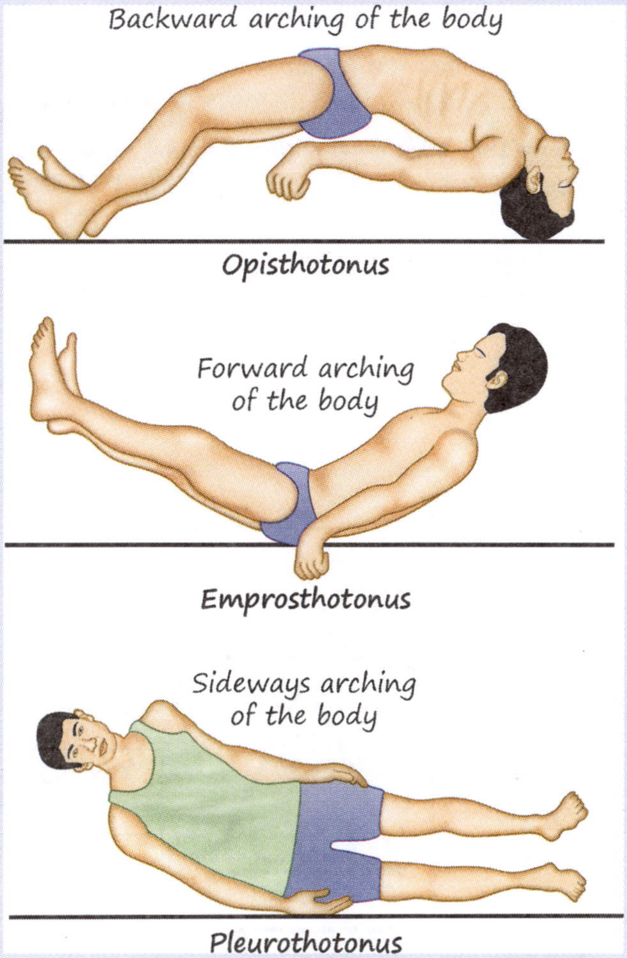

Autopsy Findings

- ***Rigor mortis: Early onset and shorter duration***[Q]*.*
- ***Postmortem caloricity***[Q]*.*

ASPHYXIANTS

Cyanide

Hydrogen cyanide (Gas)	Most rapid poison (bitter Almond smell)
Hydrocyanic acid either 2% or 4% (4% is called Scheele's acid)	
Potassium cyanide and sodium cyanide	Salts

Mechanism of Action

- *Cyanide got affinity toward ferric iron.*
- *Cyanide binds and inhibits the enzymes cytochrome oxidase and carbonic anhydrase (enzymes of cellular respiration), resulting in* ***histotoxic anoxia***[Q]*.*

Treatment

- **Hydroxycobalamin (drug of choice)**
- Nitrites (amyl nitrite and sodium nitrite)—To induce **methemoglobinemia**[Q]
- Sodium thiosulfate

Eli lilly antidote[Q]: Sodium nitrite, amyl nitrite and sodium thiosulfate

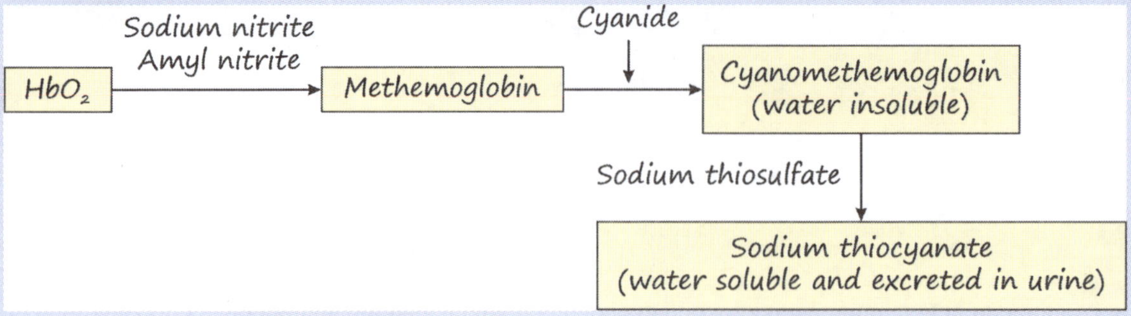

Lee Jones test[Q]: A quick bedside test that can qualitatively detect cyanide

Autopsy findings

- Bright red[Q]/ brick red[Q] postmortem staining
- Spleen is the best specimen for cyanide analysis

Carbon Monoxide

Physical Properties of CO

- Colorless
- Tasteless
- Odorless[Q] gas
- Lighter than air

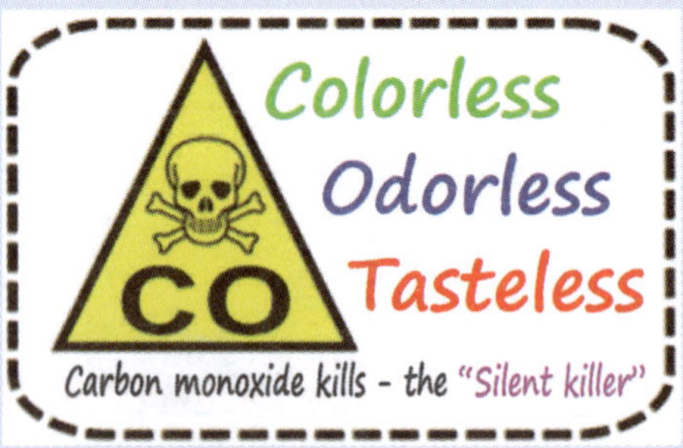

Mechanism of Toxicity

Anemic hypoxia

- It has a high affinity for Hb (about 210 times more than O_2)
- CO combines with hemoglobin to form carboxyhemoglobin producing **anemic hypoxia**[Q].

Carbon monoxide shifts the oxygen-dissociation curve to the left[Q].

Signs and Symptoms

- 0–10: No symptoms
- 10–20: Mild headache
- 20–30: Throbbing headache, emotional instability.
- 30–40: Severe headache, confusion, ataxia
- 40–50: Increasing confusion, staggering and incoordination—mistaken for drunkenness
- 50–70: Hypotension, irregular respiration, convulsions, coma and death

MANAGEMENT

1. High flow O_2
2. Hyperbaric oxygen

Tests for carbon monoxide	Autopsy findings
• Spectroscopic test • Hoppe-Seyler's test • **Kunkel's test**	Postmortem staining is **cherry red.** Skin blister present over areas like axilla, inner thigh, buttock, calves and knee. Brain Findings **Bilateral symmetrical necrosis and cavitation of basal ganglia**[Q] (globus pallidus and putamen) are the most characteristic findings.

CARDIAC POISONS

Important Cardiac Poisons

- Aconite
- Nicotine
- Digitalis
- Oleander (cerbera thevetia, cerbera odorum)

Aconite/Monk's Hood

- **Common names:** Monk's hood, mitha zaher, bish, wolf's bane, women's bane, devil's helmet or blue rocket.
- Entire plant is poisonous, however, the **root is most potent**[Q].

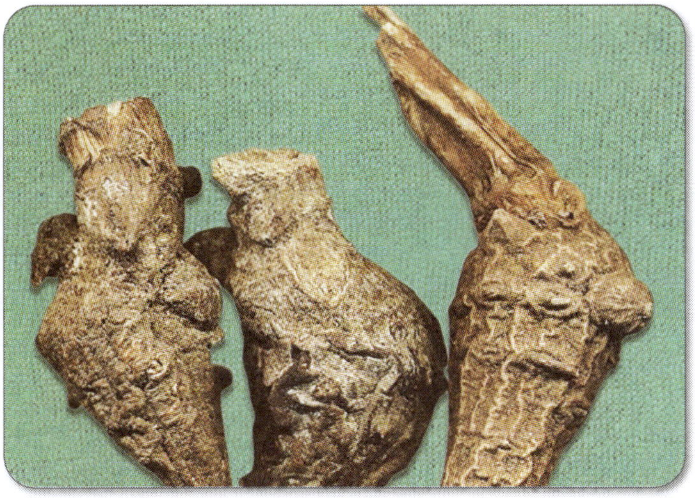

- **Active principles: Aconitine**[Q], pseudo-aconitine, indaconitine, picraconitine, mesaconitine, hypaconitine and aconine.

Clinical Features

Tingling and numbness in the mouth, tongue and pharynx[Q] (characteristic symptom of aconite poisoning)

Patients present mainly with a combination of gastrointestinal, cardiovascular and neurological features.

- **Xanthopsia:** Yellow colored halos seen around objects in vision.
- **CVS:** Bradycardia or sinus tachycardia, AV block ventricular ectopics and other arrhythmias.

Hippus

Pupillary athetosis is the rhythmic alternate contraction and dilatation of pupils.

Ideal homicidal poison[Q]

OLEANDER

Pink oleander/kaner	Yellow oleander/pila kaner
Nerium odorum	Cerebra thevetia
Active principles*** Nerin Nerioderin	Active principles*** Thevetin Thevetoxin Peruvoside Cerberin
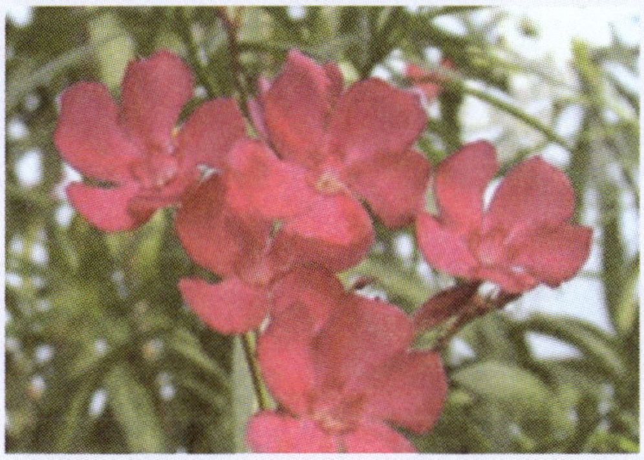	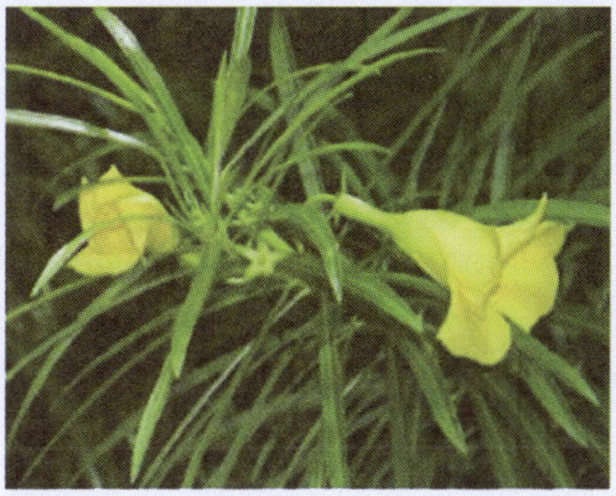

ORGANOPHOSPHATES AND ORGANOCHLORINE POISONING

Organophosphorus poisons		Carbamate	Organochlorines	Pyrethroids
Alkyl phosphates	Aryl phosphates			
• HETP, TEPP, OMPA • Dimefox, isopestox • Malathion (kill bug, Bugsoline)	• Parathion (Follidol) • Methyl parathion • Chlorthion • Diazinon (Tik 20)	Propoxur Carbaryl Baygon	• DDT, BHC (lindane) • Endrin (plant penicillin), mirex	d-allethrin, pyrethrum, allethrin, deltamethrin

Contd...

Organophosphorus poisons		Carbamate	Organochlorines	Pyrethroids
Alkyl phosphates	Aryl phosphates			
Irreversible **Inhibition of Acetylcholinesterase**[Q] (AChE)		**Reversible Inhibition of Acetylcholinesterase**[Q] (AChE)	Inactivation of Sodium channels	Inactivation of Sodium channels
Treatment: Atropine Oxime		Atropine	Symptomatic treatment and cholestyramine	Symptomatic treatment

Organophosphorus Poisoning

Cholinergic syndrome (<1 day)		Intermediate syndrome (1–4 days)	Delayed syndrome (1–4 weeks)
Muscarinic symptoms (SLUDGE BBB)	Nicotinic symptoms	Due to inadequate treatment	Distal sensorimotor polyneuropathy
S – Salivation **L** – Lacrimation **U** – Urination **D** – Diarrhea **G** – GIT upset **E** – Emesis **B** – Blurring of vision (miosis[Q]) **B** – Bronchorrhea[Q] **B** – Bradycardia	Monday – Mydriasis Tuesday – Tachycardia Wednesday – Weakness of muscles Thursday – Hypertension Friday – Fasciculations	Proximal muscle weakness Cranial nerve palsies. Neck flexor palsy.	

Diagnosis: Cholinesterase Determination in Blood[Q]

True cholinesterase (RBC)	Pseudocholinesterase (Plasma)
Correlates with clinical features and More accurate	Sensitive and commonly done

Treatment

Organophosphorus compound	Carbamates	Organochlorine
• Atropine • Oximes (diacetyl monoxime[Q] (DAM), pralidoxime (2-PAM)	Atropine	Symptomatic Rx. Cholestyramine

6. SEXUAL JURISPRUDENCE

IMPOTENCE

Males		Females	
Impotence	Inability to achieve and maintain penile erection	**Frigidity**[Q]	Decreased sexual arousal or sexual coldness
Satyriasis[Q]	Excessive sexual desire in males	**Nymphomania**[Q]	Excessive sexual desire in females

Impotence Quoad Hoc: The man is impotent toward one particular women (psychological)

Fecundation ab extra: Pregnancy that occurs in the absence of penile penetration into the vagina (by mere deposition of semen in vulva).

Virginity vs Defloration

Signs of virginity	Signs of defloration

• Breasts: Hemispherical, firm and rounded.
• Nipple: Small, areola is pink.
• Labia majora: Firm, rounded and complete.
• Labia minora: Soft, sensitive and pink in color.
• **Fourchette and posterior commissure: Intact.**
• Vaginal wall: Closely approximated.
• **Vaginal mucosa: Rugose**, reddish, sensitive to touch.
• Hymen:
  ▪ **Intact**
  ▪ Deeply situated in children and superficial after puberty
  ▪ Usually semilunar in shape.
	• Hymen: **Torn**[Q]
	• Labia majora and vagina: Loss of tone and rugosity.
	• Labia minora: Leathery and hard.
	• Fossa navicularis (will be disappeared), fourchette, posterior commissure will be torn.
	• Loss of vaginal rugosity occurs in repeated intercourse[Q]
	
	False virgin
	• Hymen is intact even after the woman has had sexual intercourse[Q]
	• Thick, fleshy or loose or elastic hymen

Location of hymenal tear

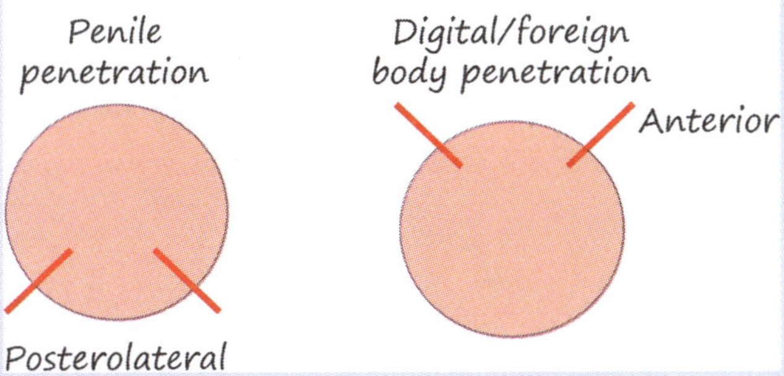

Intact hymen seen in:
- **False virgin**[Q]
- Female child (due to deep located hymen)

Types of hymen:
- Annular
- Semilunar **(mc)**
- Septate
- Cribriform
- Fimbriate: **(*The notches are commonly mistaken for hymenal tear)**

Artificial Insemination

The artificial technique of introducing semen from husband/donor into female genital tract.

Types

- Artificial insemination homologous/husband (AIH): Semen of husband used.
- Artificial insemination donor (AID): Semen of donor used.

Indications of artificial insemination	Medicolegal aspects
• Husband is impotent/sterile. • Husband is unable to deposit semen due to hypospadiasis. • Husband is suffering from hereditary disease. • Rh incompatibility between husband and wife.	**Divorce:** Done without the consent of the husband, the husband can file for divorce. **Legitimacy:** Child born out of AI is considered to be the biological child. **Adultery:** This does not amount to adultery[Q] because there is no actual physical union between the donor and the recipient. **Incest:** Remote risk of incest possible.

THE SURROGACY (REGULATION) ACT, 2021

The Act prohibits commercial surrogacy but allows altruistic surrogacy.

Surrogacy (Womb Leasing)

A surrogate mother is one, who by contract agrees to bear the child for someone else.

Types of Surrogacies

- **Commercial surrogacy:** Woman bears a child for money; she gets paid for it.
- **Altruistic/Noncommercial surrogacy:** A woman is bearing a child out of love and affection.

Eligibility for intending couple	Eligibility for surrogate mother (intending woman)
• The couple should be Indian citizens and married for at least 5 years. • They do not have any surviving child. • Live-in couples and single parents are not allowed for surrgocacy.	• A close relative of the intending couple. • A married woman having a child of her own. • Age should be 25–35-year-old. • A surrogate only once in her lifetime.

Parentage and Abortion Rules

A child born out of surrogacy will be deemed to be the **biological child** of the intending couple.

PREGNANCY, DELIVERY AND ABORTION

Pseudocyesis (Spurious/False/Phantom Pregnancy)

- Psychological disorder in which the woman falsely believes that she is pregnant, although no pregnancy exists.
- Subjective symptoms of pregnancy include abdominal distention, amenorrhea etc present; but positive signs of pregnancy are absent on obstetrical examinati on and USG.

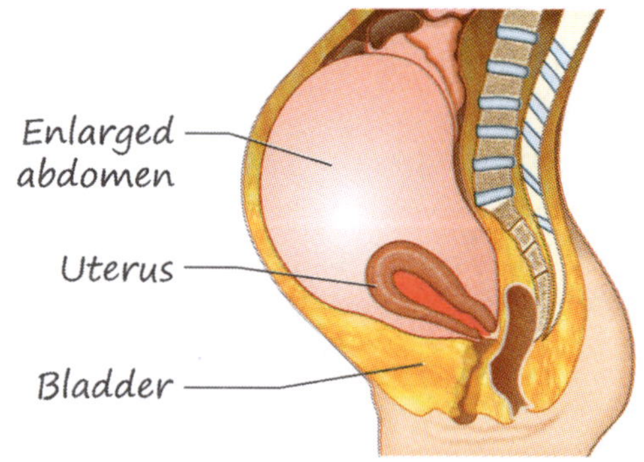

Superfecundation	Superfetation
Fertilization of two ova discharged within the **same menstrual cycle**[Q] by two different acts of coitus committed at short intervals.	Fertilization of two ova discharged from ovary at different periods of ovulation[Q].

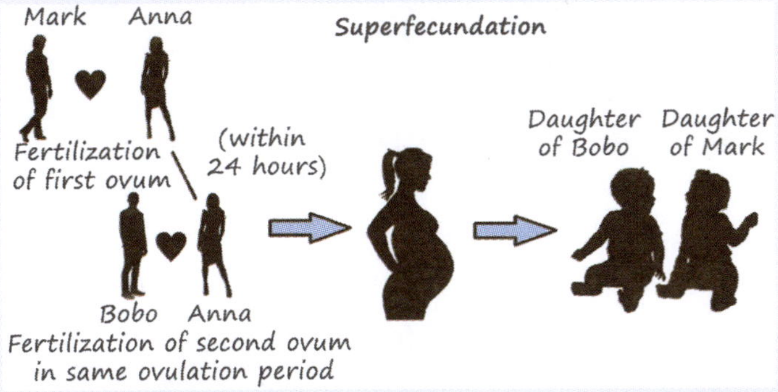

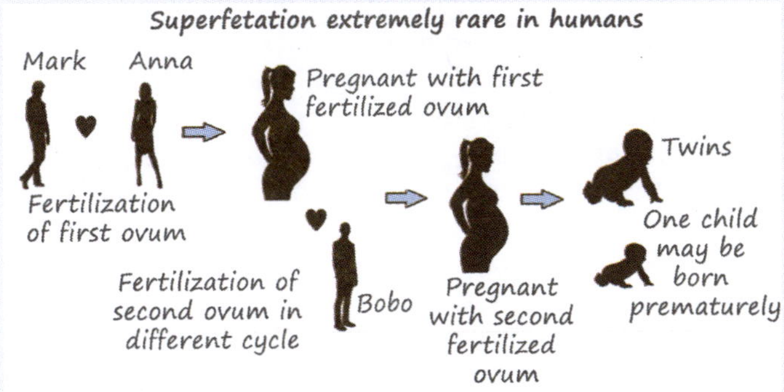

Supposititious child (fictitious child)
Woman may **pretend pregnancy**[Q] and delivery, and later produce a living child, claiming it as her own. For obtaining money or for the purpose of claiming property.
POSTHUMOUS BIRTHS: Birth of a child after the death of alleged father[Q].
ATAVISM: The child may not resemble his parents, but **resembles his grandparents**[Q].

Lochia: Alkaline discharge from uterus, a sign of recent delivery[Q]

Order of Lochia[Q]: Mnemonic—**Republic of South Africa**

R - Lochia rubra

S - Lochia serosa

A - Lochia alba

Abortion

- Medical definition: Expulsion of the products of conception up to the period of viability.
- Legal definition: Expulsion of the products of conception anytime before the full term.

Methods of Criminal Abortion (unlawful abortion).

MEDICAL TERMINATION OF PREGNANCY AMENDMENT ACT 2021

Indications[Q]:
- Therapeutic – Risk of life or grave injury to health of mother
- Eugenic – Risk of physical mental abnormalities of fetus
- Humanitarian – Pregnancy due to rape
- Social – Contraceptive failure

Consent:
Minimum age: 18 years
Minor: Guardian consent
Consent of husband: Not needed

1 Doctor opinion	**20 weeks**	**2 Doctor opinion**	**24 weeks**	**Approval from medical board**	**Term**
All indications		• Rape/incest • Minor • Mentally ill • Mass disaster times • Marital status changes (widow/divorced) • Fetal anomalies		Substantial fetal anomalies	

MTP be done anytime, in case of emergency situation.

Section 416 CrPC: If a woman who sentenced to death is found to be pregnant, the High Court shall postpone the execution, and may, if it thinks fit, commute the sentence to imprisonment for life.

VIABILITY

- Ability of the fetus to lead a separate existence after birth, by virtue of its development.
- A child is viable in 210 days (7 months).

Vagitus uterinus: Cry of the baby inside the uterus after the rupture of membranes.
Vagitus vaginalis[Q]: Cry of the baby, when the head is inside the vagina.

Live birth	Dead born
Complete expulsion of products of conception during the pregnancy and child breathes or shows any signs of life. **Signs:** • Viable child (>210 days) • Well expanded lungs • Inflammatory reaction in umbilical cord • Presence of milk in stomach	Baby died *in utero* **Signs:** • Baby shows any one of the following: ▪ Rigor mortis ▪ Maceration ▪ Mummification

Dead Born or Intrauterine Death

Maceration

Aseptic autolysis[Q]

Preconditions

- Dead child remains in the uterus for about 3–4 days
- Liquor amnii
- No air
  - **Earliest sign of maceration** is **skin slippage/reddening of skin in 12 hours after death[Q]**.
  - Joints are hypermobile.
  - **Sweetish disagreeable odor[Q]** present.

Radiological signs of maceration

Spalding sign[Q]:

- Loss of alignment and Overlapping of cranial bones of fetal skull 5–7 days after death.

Robert's sign:

- Appearance of gas shadow[Q] in chambers of heart and great vessels—as early as **12 hours.**

Ball's sign: Hyperflexion of spine is more common.

Crowding of the ribs shadow with loss of normal parallelism.

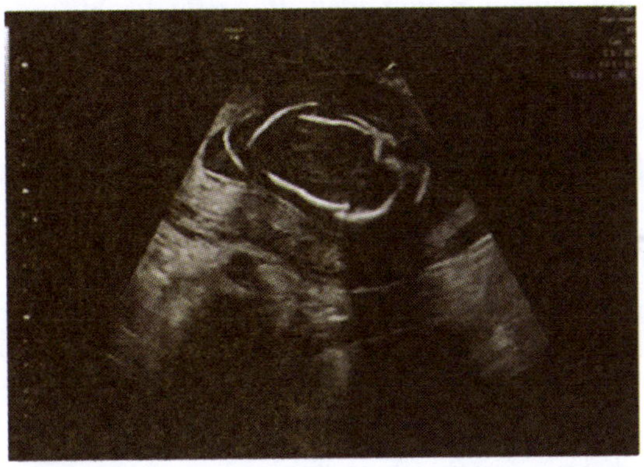

Examination of Live Born Baby

Tests for Live Birth

Level of diaphragm	In unrespired baby 3rd or 4th rib	In respired baby 5th or 6th rib
Fodere's test Checking the Weight of lungs	**30 g**	**60 g** (due to the increase in blood flow)
Plocquet test Checking the Ratio of lung weight to body weight	1:70	1:35
Wreden's test Checking the gelatinous tissue in the middle ear	**Presence of gelatinous tissue**	**Clearing of gelatinous tissue**
Breslau's second life test **Stomach bowel test** • Live born infant swallows air during respiration, and it is present in the stomach[Q] and small intestine. • The stomach and intestines are removed after tying double ligatures at each end. • They are kept under water and incision is given between the ligatures.	**No bubbles in the water**	**Bubbles in the water**
Hydrostatic test **Lung floatation test/Raygat's test** Specific gravity of lung[Q] decreases after respiration (1.040 → 0.940) The **residual air** (Not the tidal air) is tested. **Procedure** Dissect out the fetal lungs and put into a trough of water and observe. Liver is used as control.	**Lung pieces sink**	**Lung pieces float**

Battered Baby Syndrome or Caffey's Syndrome or Caffey—Kempe syndrome

Repetitive physical injuries as a result of **nonaccidental violence**[Q]
Produced by a parent or a guardian.
Slightly more in male children; Youngest or the eldest child.

Clinical Features

Multiple injuries in varying ages of healing • Fractures and injuries will be at different stages of healing. • Bruises of varying color noted.	• Most characteristic lesion-**laceration of mucosa inside the upper lip and often tear of frenulum noted.** • Slap marks, pinch Marks (butterfly bruises), six penny bruises. **CNS injuries** Infantile whiplash syndrome—shaking a child causes subdural hematoma, retinal detachment and encephalopathy.	**Radiology** **Long bones:** Metaphyseal fractureQ (so called **bucket handle fracture**[Q] **or corner fracture**): Virtually pathognomonic. **Ribs:** Nobbing fractures—multiple rib fracture in the posterior angle. **String of beads appearance**[Q] in the paravertebral gutter after callus formation **Skull fractures:** • Egg shell fractures • Depressed fracture[Q] (fracture-a-la-signature)

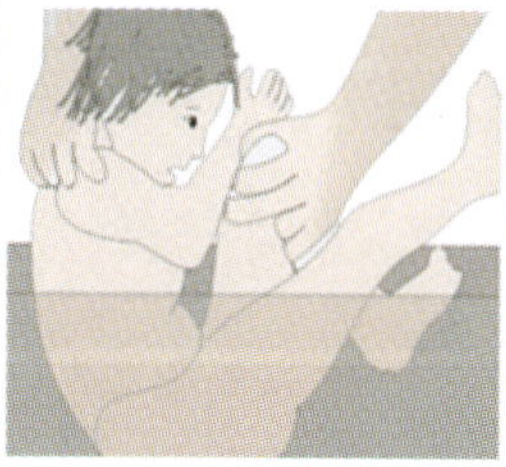
Scalds

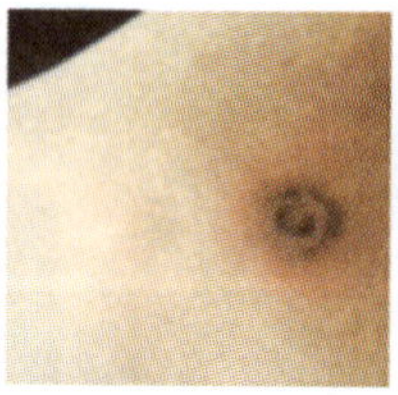
Cigarette burns

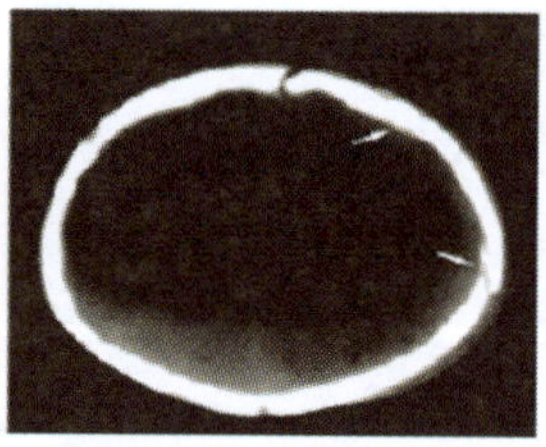
Skull fracture

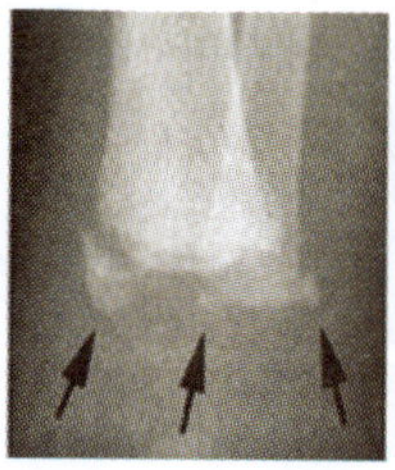
Corner fracture

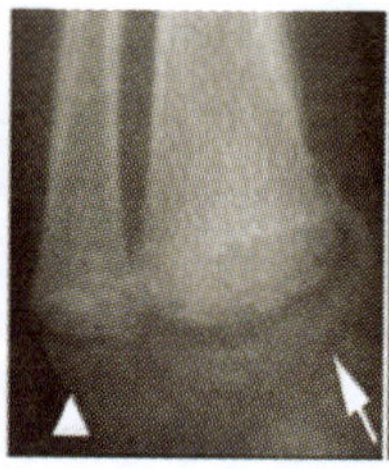
Bucket handle fracture

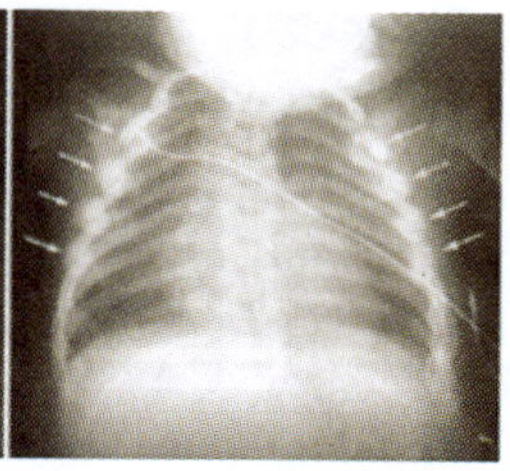
String of bead appearance

MUNCHAUSEN'S SYNDROME BY PROXY

A type of child abuse involving the parent/guardian:
- In which children are brought to doctors.
- For induced signs or symptoms of illness.
- With fictitious history.

The child is admitted frequently in the hospitals for nonexisting conditions.

SEXUAL OFFENCES

SEXUAL OFFENCE (Penile–vaginal intercourse)	SEXUAL OFFENCE (Not penile-vaginal)	PERVERSIONS/ PARAPHILIA (Sexual gratification without intercourse)	SEX LINKED OFFENCES
• Rape • Incest[Q] • Adultery[Q]	• Sodomy[Q] • Bestiality • Lesbianiasm[Q] • Buccal coitus[Q]	• Sadism[Q] • Masochism[Q] • Fetishism[Q] • Transvestic fetishism • Exhibitionism[Q] • Masturbation • Voyeurism • Frotteurism[Q]	• Indecent assault • Offences under Immoral Traffic Act

Section 375 IPC: Definition of Rape

A man is said to commit 'rape' if he:

- Penetrates his penis into the vagina, mouth, urethra or anus; or
- Inserts any object or any part of his body (not being his penis), or
- Applies his mouth into the vagina, urethra or anus; or
- Manipulates any part of her body:
  - Against her will.
  - Without her consent.
  - With her consent, when consent is obtained in fear of death or hurt or impersonation.
  - Consent given due to unsoundness of mind or intoxication or the administration of any stupefying substance.
  - With or without her consent, when she is under 18 years of age—**statutory rape.**
  - When she is unable to communicate consent.

376 IPC (1)	Punishment for rape	• **Minimum 10 years jail** • Up to life imprisonment
376 IPC (2)	• Punishment • Including custodial rape	
376 IPC (3)	• Punishment • Rape on a woman <16 years of age	

! ATTENTION: Minimum age for giving consent for sexual intercourse: 18 years[Q]
STATUTORY RAPE[Q] Sexual intercourse with a girl <18 years

Sec. 357C CrPC	All hospitals (**including private**), should provide medical treatment to the rape victims, **free of cost.** **Police intimation** to be made immediately
Sec 166B IPC	Punishment for **not treating a rape victim** in government or private hospital is punishable—1 year imprisonment
Sec 228A IPC	**Disclosing the identity** of rape victim—2 years
Sec. 327 (2) CrPC[Q]	In-camera trial in rape cases by a woman Judge/Magistrate

Medical Examination of Alleged Accused and Survivor of Rape

	Accused: Under police request 53 (A) CrPC	Accused: Under own request 54 CrPC	Victim: 164A CrPC
Consent	Reasonable force can be used	....	Mandatory

Lugol's iodine test: To detect vaginal epithelial cells[Q] on penis shaft.
Procedure:
Wipe the penile shaft with filter paper
Expose the filter paper to Lugol's iodine vapor
Result: Brown color[Q]
Time: Till 4th day[Q] after intercourse

Smegma (cheesy secretion in glanspenis):
Presence of smegma rules out possibility of complete penetration within last 24 hours It gets wiped of during complete penetration and takes 24 hours to be resecreted.

Toluidine blue test:
To detect recent micro injuries

Vaginal swabs can be taken:
Till 3 days → Spermatozoa
Till 4 days → Semen

Presence of **motile spermatozoa:** a sign of recent rape. As motility can be seen up to 6–12 hours.

Incest
Natural sexual offence between blood relations;
Not illegal in India

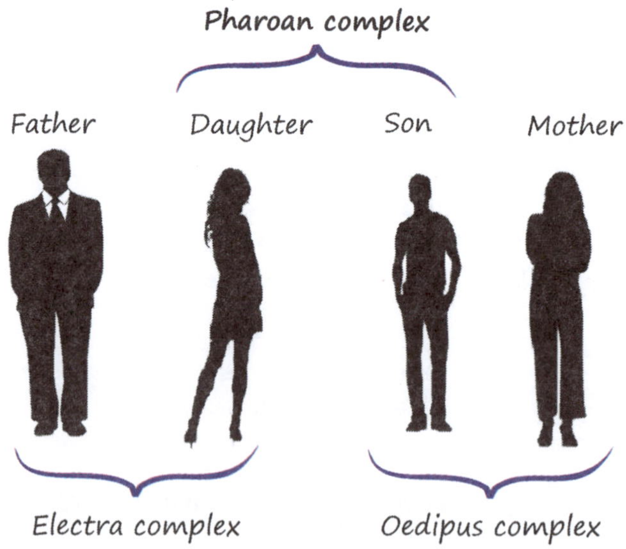

Adultery

Voluntarily having sex with someone who is not his/her legally wedded spouse.
Adultery is not a punishable crime, but if proven, adultery is a **ground for divorce.**

UNNATURAL SEXUAL OFFENCES

Bestiality, sodomy, lesbianism and buccal coitus.
Nonconsensual unnatural sexual activity is punishable under 377 IPC.

Sodomy	Tribadism/lesbianism/sapphism
Penile anal intercourse between two males or between a male and a female.	Female homosexuality[Q] by mutual acts of sexual indulgence to achieve gratification. Active lesbian is known as 'butch' or 'dyke' **Passive partner is known as 'femme'.**

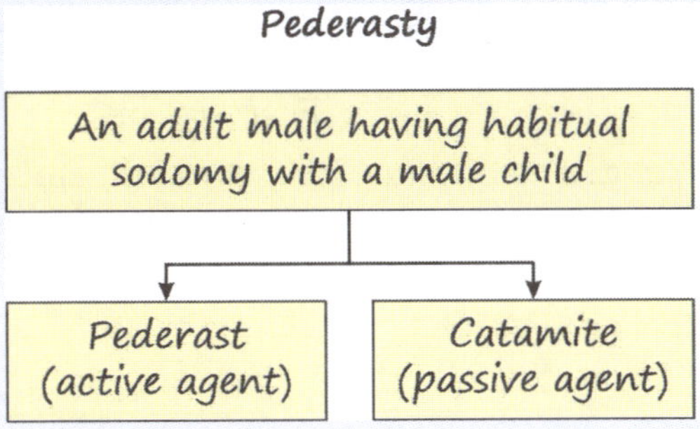

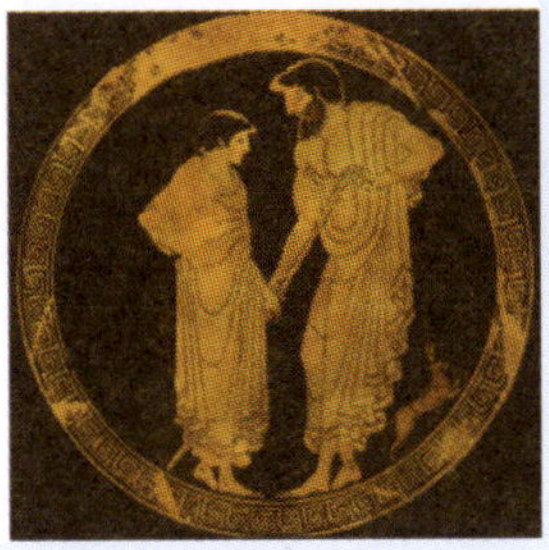

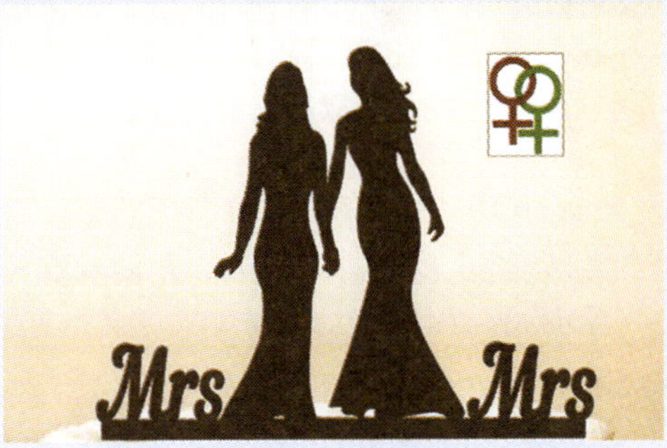

Synonyms:
Buggery
Greek Love
Pederasty: When the passive agent is a child.
Gerontophilia: When the passive agent is an adult.

Bestiality: Sexual intercourse with lower animals[Q]	**Buccal Coitus/Oral coitus/'Sin of Gomorrah'**[Q]

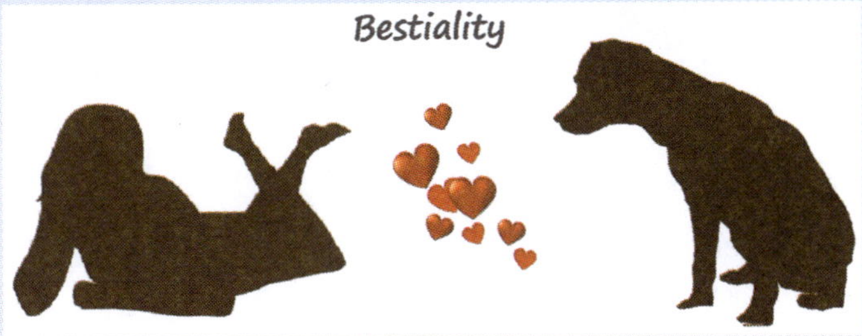

SEXUAL PERVERSIONS/PARAPHILIA

Sexual perversion is characterized by **a 6-month period of intense, recurrent sexual urges or behaviors.**

Achieving sexual gratification by	Condition
• Infliction of pain or physical cruelty on the partner. • More common in men.	Sadism[Q] Algolagnia
• Killing the partner by stabbing, slashing, mutilating the sex organs.	Lust murder
• Receiving painful stimulus from the partner for sexual pleasure. • Reverse of sadism. • More common in men.	Masochism[Q]/ Passive Algolagnia
• Having sex with the dead body.	Necrophilia[Q]
• Eating the dead body. (Eating the flesh/drinking the blood of the dead body)	Necrophagia
• Wearing the dress of opposite sex. • Desire to be identified as opposite sex.	Transvestism[Q]/ Eonism[Q]
• Exposure of genitalia in a public place to obtain sexual pleasure. • Punishable under 294 IPC.	Exhibitionism[Q]

Contd...

Achieving sexual gratification by	Condition
• Sexual arousal resulting from contact or sight of certain female parts of the body or clothing or other articles known as fetish objects. • Body parts—breasts, legs, kerchief, clothing (especially undergarments), shoes, hairs are the common fetish.	Fetishism
• Rubbing the private parts of a woman[Q] in a public crowded place.	Frotteurism[Q]
• Observing unsuspecting people undress or naked, taking bath, see the genitalia or watch intercourse to get erotic excitement and sexual gratification. • Commonly seen in males. • Voyeurs frequently peep into the bedrooms of others, and are called 'Peeping Toms'. • Punishable under 354C IPC.	Voyeurism/peeping tom/scoptophilia
• Tendency to derive sexual pleasure from the sight, thought or touch of urination (Golden showers).	Urolagnia/undinism
• Sexual gratification at sight of feces.	Coprophilia
• Sexual gratification by enema.	Klismaphilia
Sexual interest with an exclusive focus on a specific part of the body other than the genitals.	Partialism
Sexual pleasure is obtained through the compulsive use of obscene language. Making obscene telephone calls.	Scatologia
Female amputates the genitalia of the male partner.	Bobbit syndrome

SEMINAL STAIN EXAMINATION

Physical Tests for Seminal Stains

- Dried seminal stains on clothes can be examined by **UV light**[Q].
- Fluorescence noted, which is nonspecific.

Chemical Tests for Seminal Stains

Chemical tests for seminal stains
- Florence test—Choline
- Barberio's test—Spermine
- Acid phosphatase test—Acid phosphatase
- Prostate specific antigen—p30 glycoprotein
- Creatinine phosphatase test

Florence Test[Q]

Due to **choline**[Q] from seminal vesicle.

Formation of dark-brown rhombic crystals of choline iodide.

Barberio's Test[Q]

Due to the presence of **spermine**[Q] in semen.

Formation of yellow needle-shaped spermine picrate crystals.

Acid Phosphatase Test[Q]

Undiluted semen has an acid phosphatase level of 340–360 Bodansky units/mL.

A value of >100 Bodansky units with/without motile sperms indicate that ejaculation occurred within 12 hours of examination.

The levels are **not related to sperm count.**

This test is useful even in the absence of sperm.

Creatine Phosphokinase Test

CPK is high in seminal fluid and can be detected even in 6 months old stains.

Prostate Specific Antigen or Glycoprotein p30 Test

p30 can be detected in dried and old stains.

MHS – S1: Highly Reliable for Semen

Identification of Species Origin

- Precipitin test.
- LDH sss pattern (Human pattern is different from animal pattern)
- Detection of Y bodies in spermatozoa heads (which is not seen in animals).

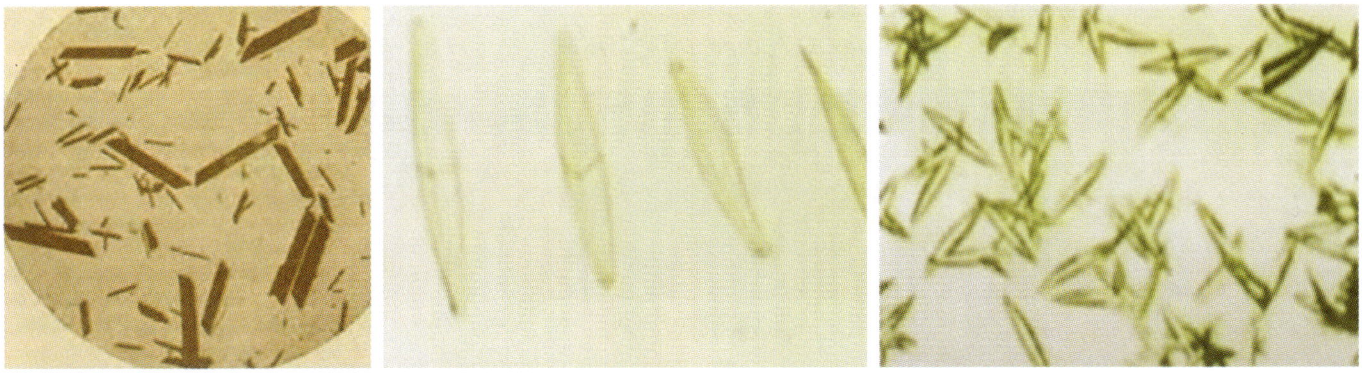

7. LEGAL PROCEDURE AND MEDICAL JURISPRUDENCE

COGNIZABLE OFFENCEOFFENSE AND NON COGNIZABLE OFFENCE

Cognizable offence—2 (c) CrPC	Noncognizable offense 2 (l) CrPC
Police can arrest a person without warrant. Example: **Rape, murder, dowry death, robbery or attempt to murder.**	Police can arrest only with warrant

INQUEST An inquest is an inquiry or investigation into the cause of death, in cases of unnatural deaths.

Types of Inquests

Inquests practiced in India	Inquests not practiced in India
• Police Inquest (most common[Q]) • Magistrate inquest[Q]	• Coroner's inquest (abolished in India on 26/6/1999 from Mumbai) • Medical examiner system (most superior) • Procurator fiscal system

Police inquest (174 CrPC)	Magistrate inquest (176 CrPC)
It is held by a police officer not below the rank of senior head constable. IO conducts an inquiry with the witnesses **(PANCHAS)** and prepares an inquiry report **(PANCHANAMA)** IO may **summon**[Q] the witnesses for inquiry (**Sec. 175 CrPC**).	See below

Magistrate inquest (176 CrPC):

Executive Magistrate (176 (1) CrPC)	Judicial Magistrate (176 (1A) CrPC)
• **Suspected** dowry deaths[Q] • Exhumation[Q]	**Custodial deaths** • Death in prison • Death in police custody[Q] • Death while under police interrogation • Death in a psychiatric hospital • Death in child reformatory schools **Suspected dowry deaths** **Exhumation**

CRIMINAL COURTS IN INDIA

Hierarchy of Indian Judiciary System and Powers of Criminal Courts

Courts	Maximum imprisonment	Fine
Supreme court judge **(Apex court National level)**	Any sentence[Q]	Unlimited
High court judge **(Apex court state level)**	Any sentence[Q]	Unlimited
Sessions Court Judge/ Additional Sessions Judge **(Apex court district level)**	Any sentence (death to be confirmed by high court[Q])	Unlimited
Assistant Sessions Judge	10 years[Q]	Unlimited[Q]
Chief Judicial Magistrate	7 years[Q]	Unlimited[Q]
I Class Judicial Magistrate	3 years[Q]	₹10000
II Class Judicial Magistrate	1 year[Q]	₹5000

Commutation of a punishment:

Any sentence awarded by a court may be enhanced or decreased by a higher court

Section 416 CrPC: The High Court shall postpone the execution of the death sentence in case of a pregnant woman, and if it thinks fit, commute the sentence to imprisonment for life.

Evidence: Statement/Document Given to Prove a Fact/Truth

Based on validity	Based on how given in court	
Direct: Directly proving the fact Example: Eye witnesses **Indirect:** Not proving the fact directly <u>Circumstantial</u>[Q]: Based on the circumstances Hearsay: Heard from someone (Invalid usually Except dying declaration)	Oral evidence **superior**[Q] than documentary evidence, as it can be subjected to **cross-examination**[Q].	Documentary evidence **Documentary evidence is accepted** by the court only after oral testimony by the person concerned. • Medical certificate • Medicolegal report • Dying declaration[Q]

Witnesse

Common witness (118 IEA) (FACT witness)	Expert witness (45 IEA)
Any person perceived the fact by his own senses. No specific age limit.	Expert in a particular field who is skilled/trained/ knowledge
Can evidence about facts. No opinions	Can evidence about facts and express opinions[Q]
1st hand knowledge rule is applicable	Not applicable

Note: Doctor can serve as both common witness and expert witness

Summons: Document compelling[Q] is the attendance of a witness in a court of law, **under penalty**[Q], on a particular day, time and place.

Subpoena: Under penalty – Willful disobedience to summon is punishable for **both civil and criminal cases.**

- Sub poena ad testificandum: To give oral evidence
- Duces tecum: To produce document related to the case.

Two summons received on same day	
One criminal court and other civil court	Attend criminal court[Q].
One lower court and other higher court	Attend higher court[Q].
Same type of courts	Attend the court from which summon is received first and inform the other court.

Conduct money (Diet Money)

It is the money paid to the witness towards the expenses in attending the court in civil cases.

- The money is paid at the time of serving the summons.
- The court fixes the amount and paid by the party calling the witness.
- **In criminal cases, no conduct money[Q]** is paid to the witness at the time of serving summons.

PROCEDURE OF RECORDING EVIDENCE IN THE COURT OF LAW

Order of Examinations[Q]: (Section 138 IEA)

Oath
↓
Chief examination (direct)
↓
Cross examination
↓
Redirect examination

OATH: "I do swear in the name of god, whatever I say shall be the truth, the whole truth and nothing but the truth."

- If person is an atheist: They can say 'I do solemnly affirm.'
- Oath is compulsory. Refusal to take oath punishable under 178 IPC.
- Exemption from oath: Child <12 years.

Sec. 191 IPC	Giving false evidence under oath (perjury definition)
Sec. 192 IPC	Fabricating false evidence
Sec. 193 IPC[Q]	Punishment for perjury

	Examination in chief (direct) by same side lawyer	Cross examination by opposite side lawyer	Redirect examination by same side lawyer
Prosecution witness	Public prosecutor	**Defense lawyer[Q]**	Public prosecutor
Defense witness	Defense lawyer	**Public prosecutor[Q]**	Defense lawyer
Leading questions Any question prompting the answer and **requiring a simple 'yes' or 'no' answer.**	**Not permitted**	**Permitted[Q]**	Not permitted

*Questions by the judge: At any time of the trial

Hostile Witness or Unfavourable Witness

- The witness who makes statement in a court contradictory to his own statement.
- **Importance:** Same side lawyer can ask leading questions.

Dying Declaration—32(1) IEA

Oral/written statement made by a dying person due to unlawful act (document used as evidence)

Procedure for Recording Dying Declaration

- Doctor has to certify "COMPOS MENTIS"
- Anyone of the following can record dying declaration
    - Magistrate (ideal)
    - Doctor
    - Police
    - Public
- No oath
- No leading questions
- Verbatim/no prompting/no alteration of words

Validity

- If the victim dies—Valid.
- If the victim survives —Invalid (only corroborative evidence).

Dying Deposition

- Judge/Magistrate → Only can record
- Accused/Defense Lawyer
- Cross-examination
- Leading questions permitted
- Oath is taken
    - **Validity:** Valid irrespective of whether the victim dies or survives.
    - Dying Deposition is superior than dying declaration.

MEDICAL LAW AND ETHICS

Medical ethics

- The moral principles which guide the members of the medical profession in their dealings with **each other, their patients and the State.**
- Self-imposed code of conduct by medical professionals.
- Violation of ethics is punishable by medical councils.

Medical etiquette

- Conventional laws of courtesy, which are followed among members of the same profession.
- Violation of ethics is not punishable.

PROFESSIONAL MISCONDUCT/INFAMOUS CONDUCT

- Disgraceful and dishonorable act by the doctors.
- Judged by other doctors[Q] of good repute.

Warning Notice (It is the list of unethical acts).

The list is incomplete, updated by SMC periodically.

Mnemonic:

Infamous conduct	B	C	D	E	F	G
6'As **A: Adultery** **A: Abortion** (criminal) **A: Alcohol** **A: Advertisement** **A: Association** **A: Addiction**	**Bribery**	**Covering** Assisting/ associating with unqualified people to carry out the work of a doctor	**Dichotomy** **'DICHOTOMY'[Q] OR 'FEE SPLITTING'[Q]** Getting commission for referring a patient to another doctor or for investigation.	Conducting active **Euthanasia**	F Issuing **False** Medical certificates	G **Gifts** Accepting gifts/cash, etc. from pharma

> **Punishments:** Given by: **State Medical Council (usually)** Appeal: **Ethic and Medical Registration Board**
>
> - Warning[Q]
> - **Penal erasure** (removal of name from medical register):
>   - Temporary[Q]
>   - Permanent erasure of name from the register is called Professional Death sentence[Q].

> **! ATTENTION:** Warning notice[Q]: List of offenses which are considered infamous conduct.
>
> Warning[Q]: Notice of caution by SMC to a doctor guilty of infamous conduct, not to repeat the offense.

PRIVILEGED COMMUNICATION

- It is an exception to professional secrecy.
- It is a statement communicated by a doctor to the concerned authority[Q].

In the interest of the community	In the interest of the patient	In the court of law
An engine or bus driver or pilot may be suffering from epilepsy, alcoholism, poor visual acuity or color blindness.	Disclosing the patient's condition and warning his relatives, in suicidal tendencies.	Doctor is bound to answer the questions, when required by the court.
A syphilitic person taking bath in public pool.		
Suspected Crime or crime, such as homicidal poisoningQ or assaultQ, the doctor is bound to report it to the nearest magistrate or police officer—39 CrPC		
Notifiable diseases like infectious diseases[Q], therapeutic abortions, epidemic and food poisoning to public health authorities.		

MEDICAL NEGLIGENCE/PROFESSIONAL MALPRAXIS

Absence of reasonable care and skill[Q] by a doctor in treating the patient, resulting in body injury or death of the patient.

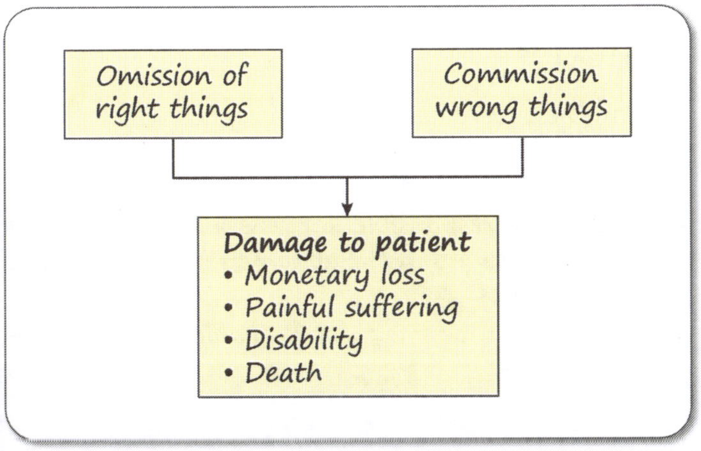

Essential Components of Medical Negligence

- D – Duty of care
- D – Dereliction of duty
- D – Damage (foreseeable/anticipated damage)
- D – Direct causation

Types of Negligence

Types	Civil negligence	Criminal negligence	Contributory negligence
Negligent act	Simple negligent act of the doctor, causing damage to the patient. **Example:** Wrong prescription[Q]. Wrong instructions.	**Gross incompetency and carelessness**[Q] in the treatment of the patient causing damage to patient. **Example:** Operation on wrong limb[Q]. Removal of wrong organ.	Negligent conduct of the patient[Q] along with doctor's negligence. **Example:** Improper history from patient. Not following doctor's instructions.
Trial court	Civil court/consumer court	Criminal court	Applies only to civil cases
Parties	Patient vs Doctor	Prosecution vs Doctor	
Burden of proof	Lies with the **patient**[Q]	Lies with the **prosecution**[Q]	Lies with the **doctor**[Q]
Punishment	Doctor should pay monetary compensation to the patient.	Imprisonment + fine. Doctor is liable under 304A IPC 336 IPC 337 IPC 338 IPC 352 IPC	Partial defense for doctor. Monetary compensation reduced.

Bolam Test

A doctor can avoid a claim for negligence if he can prove that he has provided a reasonable amount of skill and care.

VARIOUS DOCTRINES RELATED WITH MEDICAL NEGLIGENCE

Res Ipsa Loquitur[Q] **or The 'Thing Speaks for Itself**[Q]	**Doctrine of Common Knowledge**
Applicable in gross negligence. **Examples:** • Leaving surgical instruments/sponges in the abdomen. • Surgery on the wrong side/wrong organ/wrong person. • Mismatched blood transfusion. • No need of medical expert witness to prove the negligence.	Variant of res ipsa loquitur. It is based on the assumption that the negligence in the particular case is about application of common knowledge. Example: Failure to administer IV fluids in diarrhoea with dehydration. **Expert evidence is not needed.**

Calculated Risk Doctrine

- An important defense to any doctor.
- **Every medical treatment** has certain percentage of **unavoidable risks.**

Misadventure

- During treatment due to mischance/accidental damage occurring to the patient, doctor is not responsible.
- Hypersensitivity reactions caused by penicillin, tetracycline or aspirin.
- Thyroid cancer with I-131 therapy.

Novus Actus Interventions = Unrelated Action Intervening[Q]

- Any new unrelated intervening act which breaks the continuity of events and cannot be said to be an expected complication.
- Doctor is responsible for the negligent act of leaving of swabs in the abdomen in accidents and assault cases.
- Doctor may or may not be liable depending on the case.

Res Judicata ('the things have been decided')	Res Indicata (limitation period)
When the case is completed between two parties in the court, it cannot be tried again in another court between the same parties. Appeal can only be filed.	The patient should file the case against the doctor within 2 years[Q] from the date of detection of alleged negligence. Time limit applies only for civil cases to get compensation from doctor.

Products Liability

During the treatment, if the injury or the damage to the patient is due to the deficient or faulty product (drug, instrument), the manufacturer becomes responsible[Q].

Doctrine of Respondent Superior/Vicarious Liability

'Let the master answer'[Q]

An employer[Q] is responsible not only for his own negligent act, but also for the negligent act of his employees

- The chief doctor becomes responsible for any negligence of his assistants
- A hospital, as an employer, is responsible for negligence of its employees who are acting under its supervision and control.

CONSENT—(13 INDIAN CONTRACT ACT)

Types of Consent

- Implied consent: Consent implied by means of patient's gesture. (Only for physical examination).
- Expressed consent: Oral and **written (best form)**
- Blanket/open consent: Getting one consent for all the procedures in the treatment at the time of admission is legally invalid.

DOCTRINES

Doctrine of full disclosure[Q]: Complete information of the patient's condition and treatment disclosed, before obtaining consent.

Therapeutic privilege (Doctrine of partial disclosure): The doctor has the privilege of deciding how much information can be disclosed to the patient, for the benefit of the patient.

Doctrine of extended consent:

- Applicable in an unanticipated situation, where the doctor extended the consent to do additional procedures.
- Not valid in India except life-saving situations.

Loco Parentis[Q]: In an emergency involving children, when their parents or guardians are not available, consent can be taken from the person-in-charge[Q] of the child.

Doctrine of Informed Refusal: After being informed about the procedures, the patient has the right to refuse the treatment.

Rules of Consent

Age for Giving Consent

	Routine physical examination	Major procedures (like surgery, including prevaginal/ per rectal examination)
Minimum age	**12 years** For children <12 years, consent is to be obtained from a guardian (Sec. 89 IPC)	18 years

Invalid Consent

Section 90 IPC: Consent given under child <12 years, **influence, by an insane or intoxicated person is invalid**[Q]

Section 92 IPC: Emergency conditions: Consent is not required[Q] **in emergency situations, when no legal guardian is available.**

Consent in Medicolegal Examinations

Sec. 53 (1) CrPC: An accused can be examined by a doctor by using reasonable force (**without consent**), if requested by a police officer (not below SI).

Organ donation: Donation of organs **after death, the** consent from the legal guardian[Q] **is mandatory.**

Mass immunization: No need of consent[Q] required for **mass immunization**. Law provides consent for mass immunization.

Medicolegal autopsy: Consent from relatives not needed.

Pathological autopsy: Consent from relatives mandatory.

Medical Records Maintenance

Indian Medical Council (Professional Conduct, Etiquette and Ethics) Regulations, 2002

- Every physician shall maintain the medical records of **indoor patients for 3 years.**
- If any request is made either by the patients/ authorized attendant, the records shall be issued **within 72 hours.**

Declaration of Helsinki	Human research
Declaration of Oslo	Therapeutic abortion
Declaration of Tokyo (Istanbul protocol)	Torture
Geneva Convention	Medical ethics
Declaration of Malta	Hunger strikes
Declaration of Lisbon	Rights of a patient
Declaration of Ottawa	Child health

8. FORENSIC PSYCHIATRY AND BLOOD STAINS

Forensic psychiatry: It deals with the application of knowledge of psychiatry in the administration of justice.

RESPONSIBILITIES OF AN INSANE PERSON

Civil Responsibilities

Management of Property and Affairs

If the insane person is incapable of managing his property due to insanity, the court may appoint a **manager or a guardian** depending on the condition of the patient.

Consent

Consent given by an insane person is **not a valid consent**[Q].

Contract: Any contract signed by an insane person is **not valid.**

Contract signed by an insane person during the **period of the lucid interval is valid.**

Marriage

If any of the couples is proved to be insane at the time of marriage, then the marriage can be declared as '**Null and Void**[Q]'

If any one of the partners becomes insane **after marriage**, then it can be a **ground for divorce.**

Competency as a Witness in the Court of Law

An insane person is **not competent to be a witness** in a court of law, unless he/she is in a period of lucid interval.

Testamentary Capacity

The **mental ability** of a person to make a **valid will**[Q].

- **Holographic will:** A will that is written by the testator in his/her own handwriting.
  - The testator must be a **major** and of sound mind (**compos mentis**[Q]).
  - It should be **certified by a doctor.**

Criminal Responsibility of an Insane Person

McNaughten's Rule

- In India, the Criminal responsibility of an insane person is dealt with by Sec. **84 of IPC**[Q]
- An accused person is **not criminally responsible** if it is proved that, at the time of committing the crime he was suffering from such a defect of reason or from disease of mind that he did not know the nature and quality of act that he was doing.

Mnemonic

Criminal responsibility rules

Insane CAN Defend

- I: Irresistible impulse test
- C: Curren's rule
- A: American Law Institute test
- N: McNaughton's rule
- D: Durham's rule

Criminal responsibility

- **Section 84 IPC**[Q]: Act of a person of unsound mind—**not responsible**.
- **Section 85 IPC**[Q]: Act of a person by reason of intoxication caused against his will—**not responsible**.
- **Section 86 IPC**: Offense done by an intoxicated person with a particular intent to commit it—**responsible**.
- **Somnambulism**[Q] **(Sleepwalking)**: Acts done during that phase—**not responsible**[Q].

SYMPTOMS OF PSYCHIATRIC DISORDERS

Delirium

- Clouding of consciousness.
- Impaired orientation.
- Blunted critical faculties.
- Irrelevant thought content.
- Seen in high fever, drug intoxication and cerebral neoplasms.
- Such patients are not responsible for their criminal acts.

Delusion

- Disorder of **thought**[Q].
- **False belief**[Q] in something which is not a fact.
- Delusion persists even after the falsity is clearly demonstrated.

Delusion of Grandeur[Q] or Exaltation

- False belief that the person considers themselves to be powerful or wealthy that persists even when proven false.
- The person imagines himself to be very rich[Q], while in reality he may be a pauper.
- Usually seen in mania[Q].

Delusion of Persecution[Q]

- The patient imagines that he/she is going to be poisoned by his/her relatives[Q] (wife, sons or parents) or someone is going to rob his/her property.
- He/she may even commit suicide or kill his/her own family members or innocent persons in self-defense.

Delusion of Reference

He/she believes that he/she is being referred to by all agencies, media[Q] and persons around him/her in all matters (usually of negative nature) concerning him.

Delusion of Influence/Control[Q]

False belief that his thoughts, acts and emotions are influenced and controlled by external powers, like radio, hypnotism or telepathy.

Hypochondriacal Delusion[Q]

Persistent fear or belief of having a serious disease[Q] (like cancer) based on the patient's own unrealistic interpretations of physical signs and symptoms.

Delusion of Infidelity[Q]/Jealousy (Othello Syndrome[Q])

Person believes that his spouse is unfaithful, even though that is not true in reality.

Nihilistic Delusion

- The patient does not believe in his existence or the existence of earthly matters.
- Commonly seen in depression.

Fregoli Syndrome

Fregoli syndrome[Q] is a disorder in which a person holds a delusional belief that different people are in fact a single person who changes his or her appearance or is in disguise.

Erotomania[Q] (De Clérambault's Syndrome)

- Person holds a delusional belief that another person, usually of a higher social status, is in love with him/her[Q].
- It is more common in women than in men.

Hallucination: False perception[Q] without any external object or stimulus[Q].	**Phobia:** Excessive or irrational fear[Q] of a particular object or situation.
Types:	**Types:**
Visual hallucination	Fear of open spaces: Agorophobia[Q]
Auditory hallucination	Fear of closed spaces: Claustrophobia[Q]
Olfactory hallucination	Fear of heights: Acrophobia
Gustatory hallucination[Q]	Fear of darkness: Nyctophobia[Q]
Tactile/haptic hallucination[Q]: Seen in cocaine addicts[Q] (**Magnan's syndrome[Q]/Cocaine bugs**)	Fear of dirt: Mysophobia[Q]
	Fear of water: Hydrophobia

Illusion

False interpretation of a stimulus[Q], which is present.

A sane person may experience an illusion, but he is capable of correcting it with his logical thinking.

But an insane person continues to believe in the illusion even though the real facts are clearly explained.

Impulse

Sudden irresistible force[Q] compelling a person to perform the act consciously, without motive and forethought[Q].

Types

Kleptomania[Q]: Irresistible desire to steal things of little value.

Pyromania[Q]: Irresistible desire to set things on fire.

Mutilomania: Irresistible desire to mutilate animals.

Dipsomania[Q]: Irresistible desire to drink (alcohol).

Lucid Interval

It is a period during which all the signs and symptoms of insanity disappear[Q], and the person behaves normally.

Medicolegal Importance

- If he commits a crime, he is liable[Q].
- He can write a valid will[Q].
- He can testify in a court of law[Q].

Mental Health Care Act (2017)

The maximum number of days a person can be admitted on voluntary admission is 30 days, beyond which the approval of the board is necessary.

Advance directive is permitted	Prohibited procedures/practices and restrictions
Any major person can write an advanced directive related to the treatment & care in case of mental illness in future. **Importance of Advance Directive** • It is the duty of every psychiatrist to plan treatment, keeping advance directive in mind. • It will not be applicable at the time of emergency.	• No tonsuring • No compulsion to wear uniforms • **Electroconvulsive therapy (ECT):** ECT without the use of muscle relaxants and anesthesia. • ECT shall not be performed on minors. • No sterilization. • Restriction on physical restraints. • Solitary confinement is totally banned.

Attempt to Commit Suicide Not an Offense

A person who attempts to commit suicide will be presumed to be 'suffering from severe stress' and shall not be punished.

TESTS FOR BLOOD STAINS

To know the origin: human or not?	Presumptive tests Tests based on H_2O_2	Confirmatory tests
Serological tests[Q] **Precipitin test**	• Benzidine test: Blue indicates positivity. • Kastle-Meyer test or Phenolphthalein test: Pink indicates positivity	• Spectroscopy[Q] Most reliable test[Q] for detecting blood in recent and old stains • Microchemical tests **Takayama Haemochromogen Crystal Test:** Pink feathery crystals of haemochromogen. **Teichmann' Hemin Crystal Test:** Brown crystals of hemin chloride

9. LEGAL SECTIONS OF IMPORTANCE

INDIAN PENAL CODE (IPC) 1860

The various legal sections have been incorporated in the relevant sections of the chapters. The additional sections are discussed here.

Sec. 44 IPC	Injury definition

Criminal Responsibility

Sec. 82 IPC[Q]	**Criminal responsibility of person <7 years = Not liable**
Sec. 83 IPC[Q]	**Criminal responsibility of person 7-12 years = Liability depends on the mental maturity**
Sec. 84 IPC[Q]	**Criminal responsibility of insane person = Not liable**
Sec. 85 IPC	**Criminal responsibility of involuntary drunkenness = Not liable (intoxicating substance is given without the knowledge of the person)**
Sec. 86 IPC	Criminal responsibility of voluntary drunkenness = Liable (intoxicating substance is taken with intent)

Treatment of Rape Victim

Sec. 166 B IPC	Punishment for **not treating a rape victim** in government or private hospital is punishable—1 year imprisonment
Sec. 228 A IPC	**Disclosing the identity** of rape victim – 2 years

Issuing False Medical Certificates

Sec. 197 IPC[Q]	**Issuing false medical certificates—punishable offence**

Sections Related to Preservation of Evidences and Police Intimation

Sec. 201 IPC[Q]	**Causing disappearance/destruction of evidences (up to 10 years)** Suspected articles of poison to be preserved. (noncompliance—Sec. 201 IPC) **Embalming in poisoning case before autopsy**

Transmission of Fatal Infections

Sec. 269 IPC[Q]	**Negligent act likely to spread disease dangerous to life—Punishment**
Sec. 270 IPC	Willful act likely to spread disease dangerous to life—Punishment

Offences on Human Body

Sec. 299 IPC	Definition of culpable homicide not amounting to murder
Sec. 300 IPC[Q]	**Definition of murder (culpable homicide amounting to murder)**
Sec. 302 IPC	Punishment for murder—Death or Imprisonment for life
Sec. 304 IPC	Culpable homicide not amounting to murder. Imprisonment for life or 10 years and also fine.
Sec. 304 A IPC[Q]	**Death caused by rash and negligent act—2 years.**
Sec. 304 B IPC[Q]	**Dowry death—Death of a female within 7 years of marriage.**
Sec. 306 IPC[Q]	**Abetment of suicide—10 years, also fine.**
Sec. 307 IPC	Attempt to murder—10 years.
Sec. 308 IPC	Attempt to commit culpable homicide—Up to 10 years.
Sec. 319 IPC	**Definition of Hurt—Bodily pain, disease or infirmity**
Sec. 320 IPC[Q]	**Grievous Hurt—Definition**
Sec. 323 IPC	Punishment for voluntarily causing hurt—1 year, with fine.
Sec. 324 IPC	Voluntarily causing hurt with dangerous weapon—3 years also fine.
Sec. 325 IPC[Q]	**Voluntarily causing grievous hurt—7 years, also fine.**
Sec. 326 IPC	Voluntarily causing grievous hurt by dangerous weapon—10 years, also fine.
Sec. 326 A IPC[Q]	**Punishment for acid throwing (vitriolage)—Life imprisonment**
Sec. 326 B IPC	Attempt to acid throwing—5 years

Causing Harm on Provocation or Negligent Act

Sec. 337 IPC	Causing hurt by doing rash or negligent act—6 months imprisonment
Sec. 338 IPC	Causing grievous hurt by doing rash or negligent act—2 years imprisonment

Sec. 351 IPC	Assault definition
Sec. 352 IPC	Punishment for assault

Offences Against Woman

Sec. 354 A IPC	Punishment for sexual harassment (1–3 years)
Sec. 354 B IPC	Use of criminal force on woman to disrobe (3–7 years)
Sec. 354 C IPC[Q]	**Voyeurism**
Sec. 354 D IPC[Q]	**Stalking:**
	(1st offence: Cognizable and Bailable; 2nd offence: Cognizable and Nonbailable)

Sexual Perversions

Sec. 297 IPC[Q]	Necrophagia/necrophilia (1 year)

Rape and Unnatural Offences

Sec. 375 IPC[Q]	Rape – Definition
Sec. 376 IPC	Punishment for rape
Sec. 377 IPC[Q]	Nonconsensual Unnatural sexual offences—10 years

Abortion

Legal provisions against miscarriage	
Sec. 312 IPC	Punishment for causing **miscarriage**[Q]
Sec. 313 IPC	Punishment for causing **miscarriage without the woman's consent**
Sec. 314 IPC	Punishment for causing **death of the mother** by act intended to cause miscarriage
Sec. 318 IPC	Punishment for **concealment of birth**[Q] by **secret disposal of dead body**

Drunkenness

Sec. 510 IPC[Q]	Misconduct in public by a drunken person—Simple imprisonment up to 2 hours

CRIMINAL PROCEDURE CODE (CrPC) 1973

Rape Cases

IN CAMERA TRIALS—Sec. 327 (2) CrPC

GRIEVOUS HURT (SEC. 320 IPC)

- Emasculation[Q].
- Permanent privation of sight of either eye.
- Permanent privation of hearing of either ear.
- Privation of any member or joint.
- Permanent destruction of power of any member or joint.
- Permanent disfiguration of head or face.
- Fracture or dislocation of a bone or tooth[Q].
- Any hurt which **endangers life** or which causes the victim to be in **severe bodily pain**[Q], or **unable to follow his ordinary pursuits for a period of 20 days.**

Notes

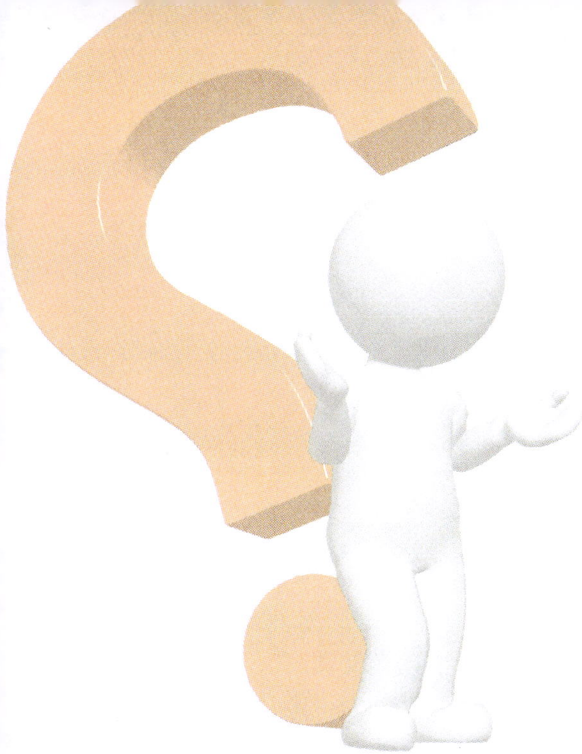

Latest Question Papers

- → NEET PG 2023
- → NEET PG 2022
- → NEET PG 2021
- → INI-CET MAY 2023
- → INI-CET NOVEMBER 2022
- → INI-CET MAY 2022
- → INI-CET NOVEMBER 2021
- → INI-CET JULY 2021
- → FMGE JULY 2023
- → FMGE JANUARY 2023
- → FMGE MAY 2022
- → FMGE DECEMBER 2021
- → FMGE JULY 2021

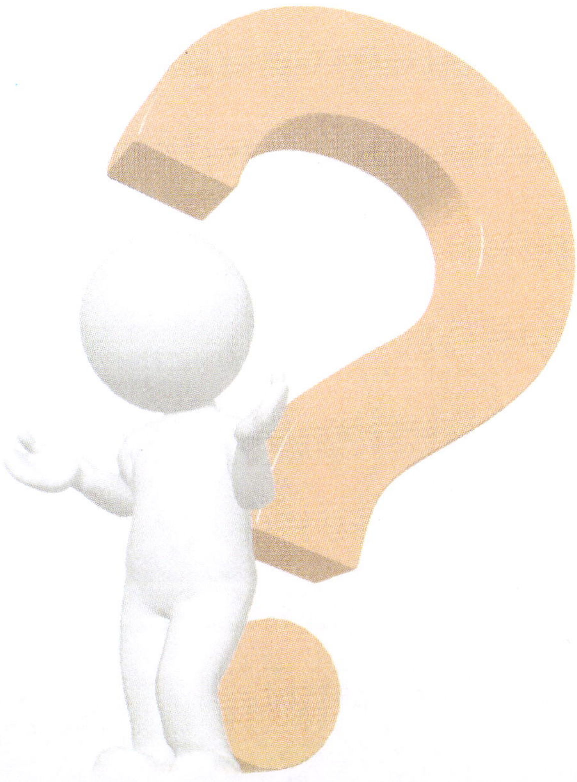

NEET PG 2023

1. 'En masse' dissection technique of autopsy where the organs removed from tongue to prostate refers to:
   a. Ghon's technique
   b. Letulle's technique
   c. Virchow's technique
   d. Rokitansky's technique

Ans. b. Letulle's technique

2. The technique of autopsy used in cases of HIV infected dead body is:
   a. Ghon's
   b. Letulle's
   c. Virchow's
   d. Rokitansky's

Ans. d. Rokitansky's

3. A laborer while working under hot sun collapsed with loss of consciousness and brought to the emergency department. On examination, his body temperature was found to be 106°F. The least likely finding is:
   a. Hypotension
   b. Tachycardia
   c. Hot skin
   d. Sweating

Ans. d. Sweating

4. Section 314 of IPC deals with:
   a. Causing miscarriage with the consent of the mother
   b. Causing miscarriage without the consent of the mother
   c. Causing death of the mother by miscarriage
   d. Causing death of quick unborn child while trying to kill mother

Ans. c. Causing death of the mother by miscarriage

5. A dead body is brought to the mortuary. On external examination, rectal temperature was found to be 39°C. The probable cause could be:
   a. Intraabdominal hemorrhage
   b. Septicemia
   c. Corrosive poisoning
   d. Cyanide poisoning

Ans. b. Septicemia

6. A child has been brought by the police to the dept. of Forensic Medicine. Examination revealed reddening around the anus with tenderness during examination. Laboratory examination of anal swab by using picric acid reagent showed yellow needle shaped crystals under microscope. The test conducted is:
   a. Teichmann's test
   b. Takayama test
   c. Florence test
   d. Barberio's test

Ans. d. Barberio's test

7. A playing child, plucked the fruit from a plant and consumed it. The child was brought to hospital with painful swallowing, photophobia, inability to pass urine and hyperthermia. The poison and the antidote in this case are:
   a. Datura and physostigmine
   b. Datura and pralidoxime
   c. Yellow oleander and physostigmine
   d. Yellow oleander and pralidoxime

Ans. a. Datura and physostigmine

8. After consuming some seed, a 45-year-old man presented to the emergency room with generalized muscular spasm and backward arching. The probable seed she had consumed is/are:
   a. Datura seeds
   b. Strychnos nux vomica
   c. Abrus precatorius
   d. Ricinus communis

Ans. b. Strychnos nux vomica

9. A poor farmer with history of successive crop failure develops progressive spastic paraparesis, upper motor neuron signs, and unstable gait. The toxin responsible is:
   a. Beta-N-oxalyl amino-L-alanine (BOAA)
   b. Aflatoxin
   c. Strychnine
   d. Ergotoxine

Ans. a. Beta-N-oxalyl amino-L-alanine (BOAA)

10. The hyperthermia associated with the treatment of organophosphorus compounds poisoning with atropine and pralidoxime is due to:
   a. OPC poison
   b. Atropine toxicity
   c. Oximes toxicity
   d. Aspiration pneumonia

Ans. b. Atropine toxicity

11. A chronic alcoholic patient develops confusion, ophthalmoplegia and ataxia. The diagnosis is:
   a. Delirium tremens
   b. Wernicke's encephalopathy
   c. Korsakoff's psychosis
   d. Paranoia

Ans. c. Korsakoff's psychosis

12. In case of aspirin poisoning of 100 tablets, which treatment modality is useful:
   a. N-Acetyl cysteine
   b. Alkaline diuresis by IV $NaHCO_3$
   c. Gastric lavage with $NaHCO_3$
   d. Flumazenil

Ans. b. Alkaline diuresis by IV $NaHCO_3$

13. A farmer while sleeping in his field, felt something bit him. He saw something moving away. He presents to hospital with pain at the site, with excessive bleeding. This is suggestive of bite due to:
   a. Scorpion sting
   b. Cobra bite
   c. Viper bite
   d. Wasp sting

Ans. c. Viper bite

NEET PG 2022

14. A female has come to gynecologist for hysterectomy. The doctor explains the benefits and risks of the procedure and obtained consent. This consent is known as:
   a. Implied consent
   b. Informed consent
   c. Blanket consent
   d. Opt out consent

Ans. b. Informed consent

15. A doctor who is drunk, while performing the surgery, injured a major vessel causing death of patient. This is:
   a. Civil negligence
   b. Criminal negligence
   c. Therapeutic misadventure
   d. Dichotomy

Ans. b. Criminal negligence

16. The injury is suggestive of:

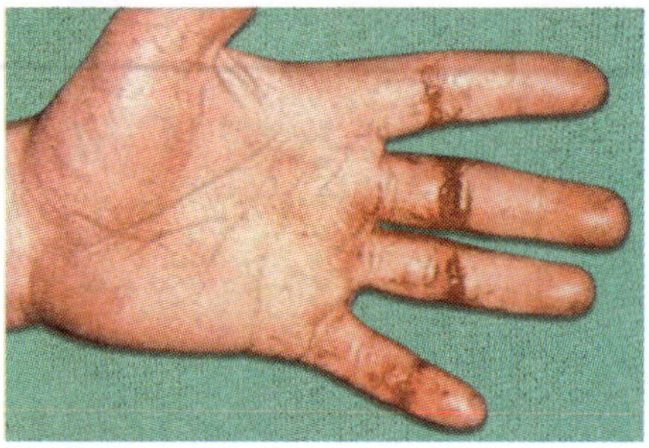

   a. Postmortem wound
   b. Self-inflicted cuts
   c. Defense cuts
   d. Hesitation cuts

Ans. c. Defense cuts

17. This type of hymen is:

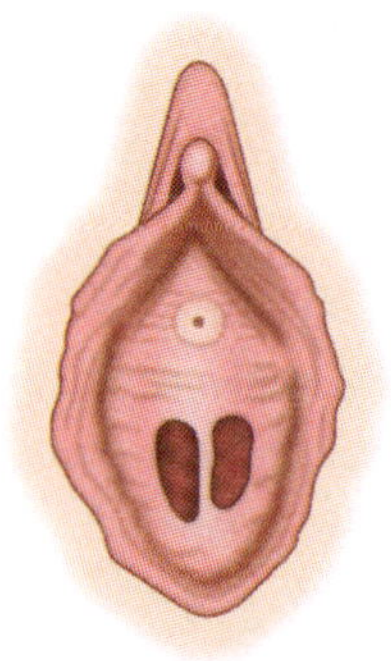

   a. Septate b. Fimbriated
   c. Annular d. Semilunar

Ans. a. Septate

18. A patient has been brought to emergency with respiratory depression, pin point pupil and in comatose condition. The antidote to be given is:
   a. Naltrexone b. Naloxone
   c. Flumazenil d. Oximes

Ans. b. Naloxone

19. Identify the range:

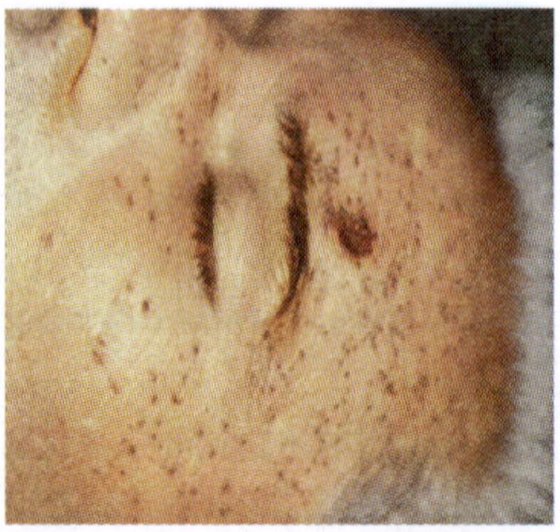

a. Pistol intermediate range
b. Rifle close range
c. Pistol close range
d. Shot gun intermediate

Ans. a. Pistol intermediate range

20. A 45-year-old male came with acute loss of hair in head and madarosis. The wife had given history of behavioral changes. The doctor examined the nails and made the diagnosis. The condition is:
a. Arsenic poisoning
b. Thallium poisoning
c. Mercury poisoning
d. Lead poisoning

Ans. b. Thallium poisoning

21. A 3-year-old child brought to hospital with history of consumption of iron tablets. History of abdominal pain, diarrhea and vomiting. The child is in comatose condition. The treatment is:
a. Desferrioxamine
b. BAL
c. Activated charcoal
d. Penicillamine

Ans. a. Desferrioxamine

22. A girl had been brought with history of excessive consumption of paracetamol tablets. The treatment to be given is:
a. N acetyl cysteine
b. Naloxone
c. Flumazenil
d. Atropine

Ans. a. N acetyl cysteine

23. A dead body is brought with ligature mark over neck, which is encircling the neck, transverse, below the thyroid cartilage. No salivary dribbling noted. This condition is:
a. Throttling
b. Mugging
c. Ligature strangulation
d. Hanging

Ans. c. Ligature strangulation

24. In a case of lead poisoning, the enzymes inhibited are:
a. ALA synthase
b. Uroporphyrinogen III synthetase
c. Ferrochelatase
d. Coproporphyrinogen reductase

Ans. c. Ferrochelatase

25. A 10-Year-old child with burns involving the front of right upper limb, front of right side of the chest, front of right side of abdomen and front of right leg. The percentage of burns involved is:
a. 5–10%
b. 15–20%
c. 25–30%
d. 35–40%

Ans. b. 15–20%

26. In a court trial, leading questions are not permitted in all of the following; except:
a. Re-examination
b. Cross examination
c. Dying declaration
d. Direct examination

Ans. b. Cross examination

NEET PG 2021

27. Identify the injury:

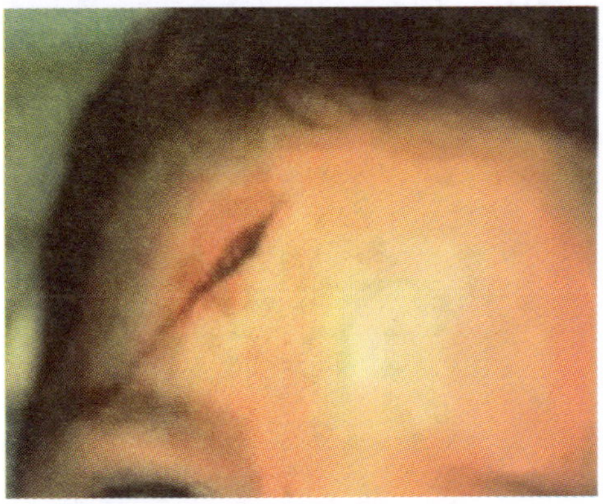

a. Incised looking laceration
b. Incision
c. Lacerated looking incision
d. Laceration

Ans. a. Incised looking laceration

28. While recording evidence in the court of law, the lawyer asked the witness 'Did A killed B?'. Witness said 'Yes'. This type of question is permitted in:
a. Examination-in-chief
b. Direct examination
c. Re-examination
d. Cross examination

Ans. d. Cross examination

29. Not suggestive of cocaine poisoning is:
a. Bradycardia
b. Hyperthermia
c. Agitation
d. Incoordination

Ans. a. Bradycardia

30. Active principle of this seed is:

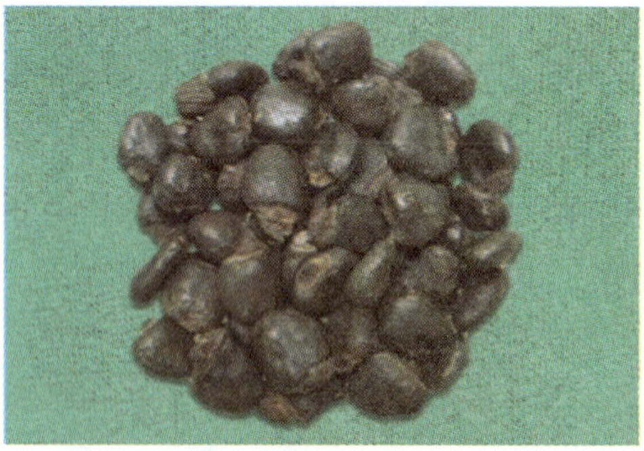

a. Ricin
b. Crotin
c. Abrin
d. Bhilawanol

Ans. d. Bhilawanol

31. True regarding the change seen in this image is:

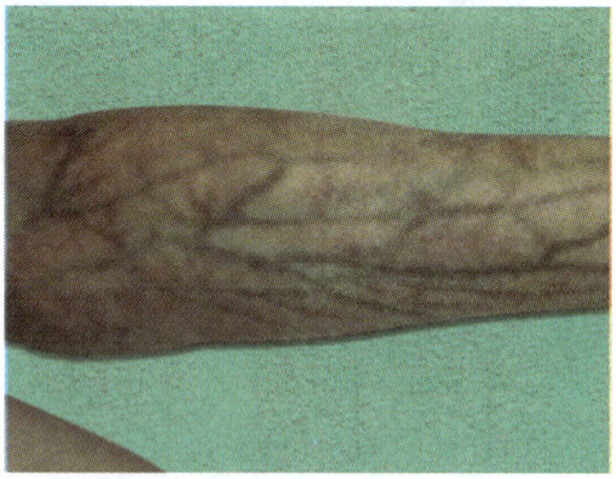

a. Due to vascular disease
b. Due to sulfhemoglobin
c. Due to nonbacterial cause
d. Seen within 24 hours after death

Ans. b. Due to sulfhemoglobin

32. This phenomenon is due to:

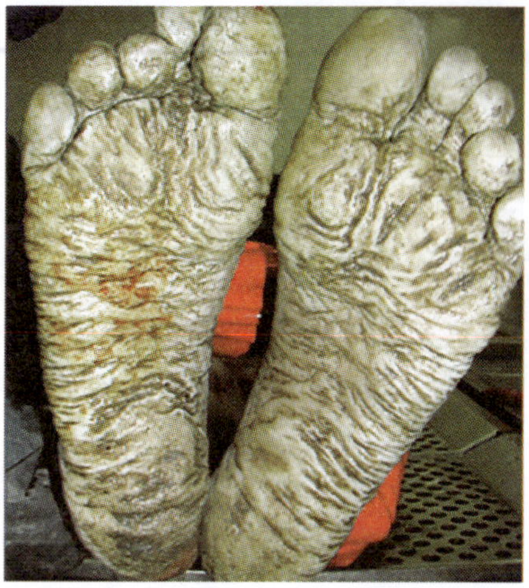

a. Case of torture in hot water
b. Case of postmortem hanging
c. Case of immersion in water for 36 hours
d. Case of falanga

Ans. c. Case of immersion in water for 36 hours

33. Wife gave birth to twins. The suspicious husband underwent DNA typing, where he found out that he was not the father of one of the twins. Such cases are known as:
a. Superfetation
b. Superfecundation
c. Papyraceous child
d. Supposititious child

Ans. b. Superfecundation

34. A person was sitting naked in the balcony facing a crowded park and getting sexual gratification. This paraphilia is known as:
a. Voyeurism
b. Exhibitionism
c. Masochism
d. Fetishism

Ans. b. Exhibitionism

35. A man was working in field, collapsed in a hot summer afternoon. Which of the following symptoms is least likely to be seen?
a. Sweating
b. Disorientation
c. Hot skin
d. Tachycardia

Ans. a. Sweating

36. A child consumed some unknown fruit. After some time, he started symptoms of irritability, restlessness, confusion, inability to pass urine, hot skin and photophobia. Select the poison and antidote:
   a. Datura and physostigmine
   b. Yellow oleander and physostgmine
   c. Datura and digibond
   d. Yellow oleander and digibond

Ans. a. Datura and physostigmine

INI-CET MAY 2023

37. Which of the following is not true about postmortem changes?
   a. Greenish discoloration in Right iliac fossa is the earliest sign of decomposition
   b. In drowning postmortem hypostasis is seen in lower limbs
   c. Adipocere is seen in bodies recovered from water source
   d. Cadaveric spasm is seen only in specific group of muscles

Ans. b. In drowning postmortem hypostasis is seen in lower limbs

38. Blackfoot disease is an endemic peripheral vascular disease seen in toxicity of which of the following metal?
   a. Antimony
   b. Arsenic
   c. Barium
   d. Cadmium

Ans. b. Arsenic

39. A female was brought for autopsy with alleged history of being found at the lake in village. All of the following are suggestive of antemortem drowning; EXCEPT:
   a. Water in stomach
   b. White leathery foam around mouth and nostrils
   c. Positive diatom test
   d. Washerwoman hands and feet

Ans. d. Washerwoman hands and feet

40. A 12-year-old girl is brought by lady police sub-inspector with alleged history of sexual violence 2 days back. She was accompanied by her mother. The registered medical practitioner should do which of the following as the next step?
   a. Preserve clothing
   b. Take consent for genital examination
   c. Take a detailed history
   d. Documentation of injuries and examination findings

Ans. c. Take a detailed history

41. A 5-year-old boy went to temple in a village with his grandmother. He was crying inconsolably on the way back. He was taken to the emergency department within 3 hours. He had altered sensorium, cold clammy extremities, increased salivation and excessive sweating. On examination he was pale, had priapism with the following vitals: BP—140/78 mmHg, HR—152/min, RR—36/min sPO2 of 96%. Which of the following would you use in management?
   a. Anti-snake venom
   b. Methylprednisolone
   c. Adrenaline
   d. Prazosin

Ans. d. Prazosin

42. During the examination of a drunkard, he smells of alcohol and has red conjunctiva. But his motor coordination is normal, he can walk in a straight line and can talk normally. Which of the following is true?
   a. He has consumed alcohol
   b. He has consumed alcohol but is not under its influence
   c. He has consumed alcohol and is under the influence of alcohol
   d. He has not consumed alcohol

Ans. b. He has consumed alcohol but is not under its influence

43. Identify the following:
   (The patient having burns with blisters with surrounding hyperemia in the chest and abdomen.)
   a. Blister due to barbiturate poisoning
   b. Blister due to antemortem burns
   c. Edema due to chemical burn
   d. Pemphigus vulgaris

Ans. b. Blister due to antemortem burns

44. In a death due to firearm injury, the entry wound only shows abrasion collar. The range of firearm is:
a. Contact range b. Close range
c. Near range d. Distant range

Ans. d. Distant range

45. Formication or magnan symptom is seen in:
a. Cocaine b. Cannabis
c. Opium d. MDMA

Ans. a. Cocaine

46. Which of the following is not a part of Right slogan for snake bite treatment?
a. Reassure b. Incision
c. Get to hospital d. Immobilization

Ans. b. Incision

47. A 29-year-old woman is brought into the emergency department by the police due to being found unresponsive in the park. At the scene, an empty syringe was found. Her respirations are 6/min. Physical exam is significant for depressed mental status, bilateral track marks, and miotic pupils. Antidote is ?
a. Naloxone b. Atropine
c. Pethidine d. Methadone.

Ans. a. Naloxone

INI-CET NOVEMBER 2022

48. A patient with previous history of abdominal surgery comes to hospital with abdominal pain and fever. X-ray of abdomen is shown below. This corresponds to:

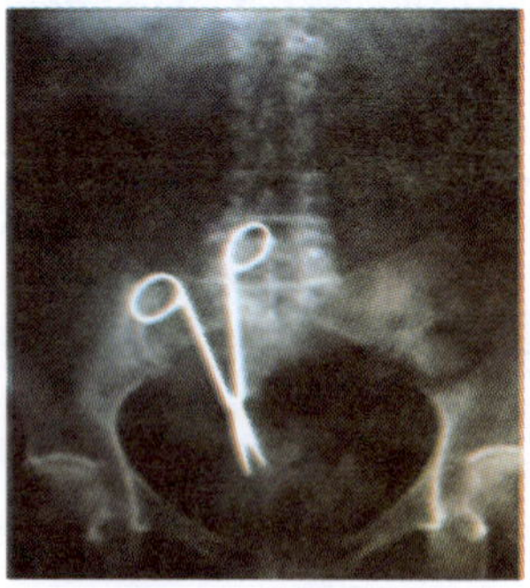

a. Res ipsa loquitur
b. Res Judicate
c. Novus actus interveniens
d. Vicarious liability

Ans. a. Res ipsa loquitur

49. Dead body of a child was recovered from a river with froth around the mouth and nostrils. Froth was oozing out even after wiping it. The postmortem finding not seen in such scenario is:
a. Ballooning of lungs
b. Cadaveric spasm of hands with mud in closed fist
c. Paltauf's hemorrhages
d. Arsenic from hair sample

Ans. d. Arsenic from hair sample

50. In a firearm injury, tattooing is noted around the wound of entry. The cause for tattooing is:
a. Hot air and flame
b. Muzzle of the gun
c. Unburnt gunpowder particles
d. Smoke

Ans. c. Unburnt gunpowder particles

51. Spanish windlass technique, is also known as a type of:
a. Bansdola b. Mugging
c. Throttling d. Garroting

Ans. d. Garroting

52. Match the teeth with age of their eruption:

A. Lateral incisor	1. 6–7 years
B. Canine	2. 8–9 years
C. First molar	3. 11–12 years
D. Third molar	4. 18–25 years

a. A-1, B-3, C-2, D-4
b. A-2, B-3, C-1, D-4
c. A-1, B-2, C-4, D-3
d. A-3, B-2, C-1, D-4

Ans. b. A-2, B-3, C-1, D-4

53. Match the following plant poisons with their active principles:

A. Opium	1. Abrine
B. Nux vomica	2. Morphine
C. Datura	3. Hyoscyamine
D. Abrus precatorius	4. Brucine

a. A-1, B-2, C-3, D-4
b. A-1, B-3, C-2, D-4
c. A-2, B-4, C-3, D-1
d. A-1, B-2, C-4, D-3

Ans. c. A-2, B-4, C-3, D-1

54. Which of the following is not a cardiac toxin?

a. Atropa belladonna b. Aconite
c. Cerbera thevetia d. Digitalis

Ans. a. Atropa belladonna

55. A 70-year-old lady with an alleged history of impact on head following fall on a ice slab presents to the ER after 4 days with symptoms of headache, nausea, excessive sleep and lethargy. CT scan showed a crescent shaped hyper density crossing the sutural lines. She died after 4 days. What is the finding in the depicted image?

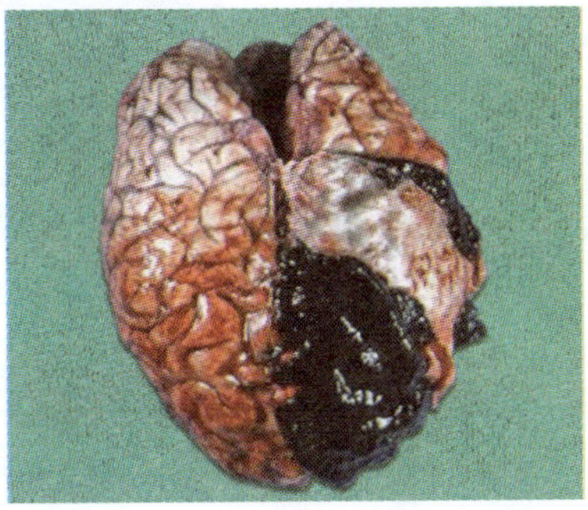

a. EDH b. SDH
c. SAH d. ICH

Ans. b. SDH

56. The below given picture depicts:

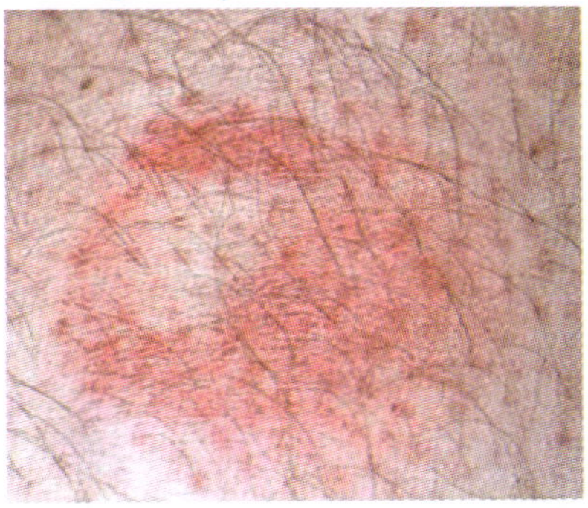

a. Incision b. Contusion
c. Laceration d. Stab wound

Ans. b. Contusion

57. Identify the finding in image:

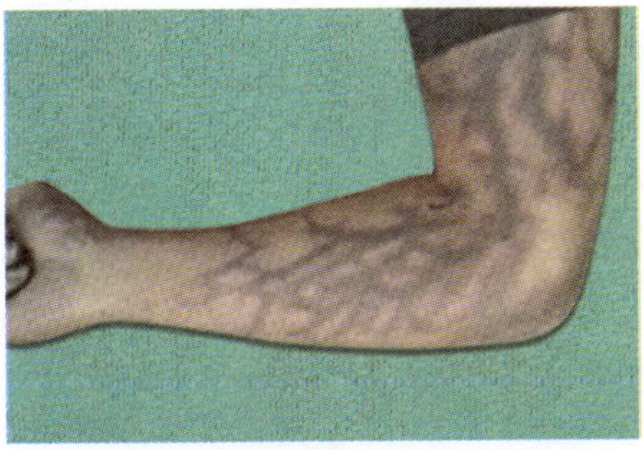

a. Postmortem lividity
b. Marbling
c. Tattooing
d. Ecchymosis

Ans. b. Marbling

58. Hooch tragedy is due to the consumption of:

a. Ethanol b. Methanol
c. Ethylene glycol d. Isopropyl alcohol

Ans. b. Methanol

59. A pregnant woman visited an obstetrician with a history of absent fetal movements. USG revealed gas shadow in the aorta. This sign is known as:

a. Spalding's sign b. Deuel's Halo sign
c. Ball sign d. Robert's sign

Ans. d. Robert's sign

60. Match the following:

A. Exhibitionism	1. Rubbing the genitalia to opposite sex
B. Frotteurism	2. Wearing clothes of opposite sex
C. Eonism	3. Sexual intercourse with dead bodies
D. Necrophilia	4. Exposing the private parts in public

a. A-4, B-1, C-2, D-3
b. A-1, B-3, C-2, D-4
c. A-2, B-4, C-3, D-1
d. A-1, B-2, C-4, D-3

Ans. a. A-4, B-1, C-2, D-3

61. If the cry of a fetus is heard in vagina before the complete delivery, it is known as/due to:

a. Vagitus vaginalis
b. Infection of vagina
c. Infection of uterus
d. Infection of both vagina and uterus

Ans. a. Vagitus vaginalis

62. First aid and hospital management for snake bite envenomation is:

A. Kill the snake
B. Immobilization
C. Wash the wound
D. Incision and suction

E. Application of tourniquet
F. Administration of ASV
a. A, C and D b. B, C and D
c. B, C and E d. B and F

Ans. d. B and F

INI-CET MAY 2022

63. Ridge pattern of fingerprints appears between:
a. 26 to 28 weeks of intrauterine life
b. 12 to 16 weeks of intrauterine life
c. 24 to 28 weeks of intrauterine life
d. 32 to 36 weeks of intrauterine life

Ans. b. 12 to 16 weeks of intrauterine life

64. In chronic arsenic poisoning following clinical features are present:
1. Aldrich – mees line over the nails
2. Raindrop type of pigmentation resembles fading measles rash
3. Mixed neuropathy (motor + sensory)
4. Luminescent vomitus
5. Bone marrow depression

a. 1, 2, 3, 5
b. 1, 2, 3, 4, 5
c. 1, 2, 3
d. 1, 2, 4, 5

Ans. a. 1, 2, 3, 5

65. Identify the mechanical injury given in the picture:

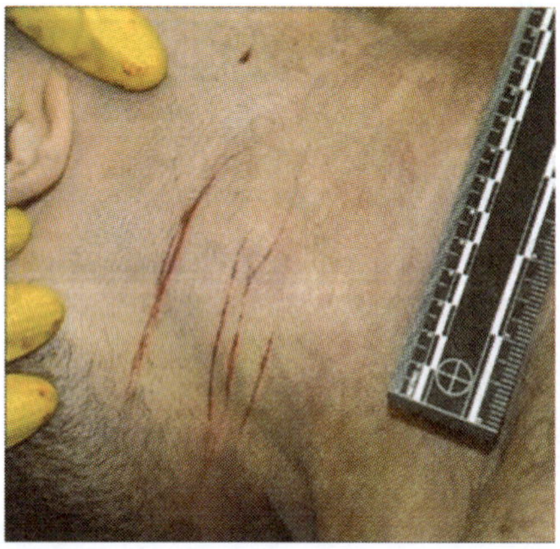

a. Graze abrasion
b. Hesitation cuts
c. Six penny bruise
d. Patterned abrasion

Ans. b. Hesitation cuts

66. Following is used to identify the vaginal cells on glans penis during the examination of accused of rape:
a. Precipitin test
b. Florence test
c. Lugols iodine
d. Toludine blue

Ans. c. Lugols iodine

67. Identify the poisonous plant having yellow flowers and seeds contained in pricky capsules:

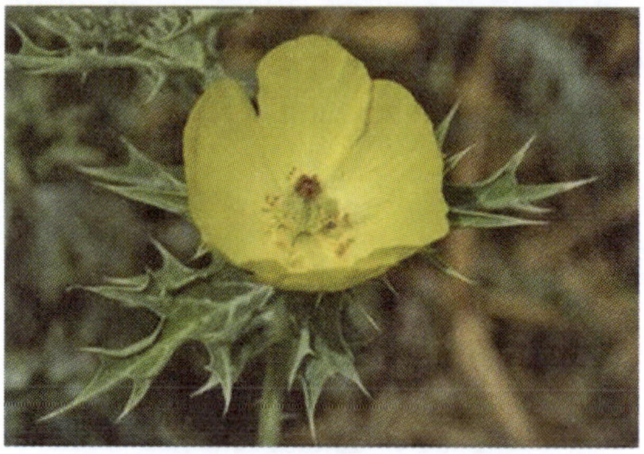

a. Argemona mexicana (sialkanta)
b. Nerium odorum
c. Papaver somniferum
d. Calotropis procera

Ans. a. Argemona mexicana (sialkanta)

68. Treatment of acute arsenic poisoning:
a. Dialysed iron
b. Freshly prepared hydrated ferric oxide
c. CA EDTA
d. Dimercaprol or BAL

Ans. d. Dimercaprol or BAL

69. In case of alleged murder of Mr A by Mr B at a certain place on a particular day and time, Mr C saw Mr B with a knife on that day at that place a few minutes before the murder. This is _____ evidence?
a. Direct evidence
b. Indirect evidence or circumstantial evidence
c. Hearsay evidence
d. Hostile witness

Ans. b. Indirect evidence or circumstantial evidence

70. Following are muscarinic manifestations of organophosphorus poisoning; except:

a. Urinary incontinence and diuresis
b. Bradycardia
c. Mydriasis
d. Bronchoconstriction and PUL

Ans. c. Mydriasis

71. Which of the following is not the feature of cocaine intoxication?
a. Tingling and numbness of hands and feet
b. Constricted pupil and bradycardia
c. Hypertension
d. Hyperthermia

Ans. b. Constricted pupil and bradycardia

72. A 27-year-old comes to emergency with salivation, diarrhea, watery eyes, dysuria. What will be first line of management?
a. IV calcium gluconate
b. Atropine
c. Pralidoxime
d. Obidoxime

Ans. b. Atropine

73. Most characteristic feature of muscarinic symptoms in organophosphorous poisoning among the following:
a. Respiratory symptoms like salivation, rhinorrhea, bronchorrhea and bronchospasm
b. Mydriatic pupil
c. Bradycardia
d. Skeletal muscle contraction

Ans. a. Respiratory symptoms like salivation, rhinorrhea, bronchorrhea and bronchospasm

74. Which of the following causes hypertension?
a. Cocaine
b. Acute alcoholism
c. OP poison
d. Acute arsenic poisoning

Ans. a. Cocaine

INI-CET NOVEMBER 2021

75. A 49-year-old male is brought to emergency after a bomb explosion. He has multiple abrasions and lacerations injuries at right side chest and abdomen. Which of the following is responsible for proximity of these injuries?
a. Falling masonry b. Barotrauma
c. Flying missiles d. Burns by fire

Ans. c. Flying missiles

76. A person is brought to emergency dept, with laceration on the forehead and back of head. Mechanism of such laceration on forehead is by?
a. Skin crushed between 2 hard objects
b. Shearing force
c. Semi sharp objects
d. Over stretching

Ans. a. Skin crushed between 2 hard objects

77. A dead body with an alleged history of suicide by hanging is brought to mortuary for autopsy. On external examination, there was a ligature mark covering about one-third of the circumference of neck, salivary stain, dilated pupils and opened right eye and closed left eye. The reason for opened right eye is:
a. Compression of carotid artery
b. Compression of internal jugular vein
c. Compression of cervical sympathetic chain
d. Compression of vagus nerve

Ans. c. Compression of cervical sympathetic chain

78. The mechanism of action of Organophosphorus compounds on Acetylcholine esterase is by:
a. Competitive inhibition
b. Noncompetitive inhibition
c. Reversible competitive inhibition
d. Irreversible competitive inhibition

Ans. d. Irreversible competitive inhibition

79. A pelvis is brought to the forensic department for sex determination. The doctor had opined as Male pelvis based on following findings:
A. 'U' Shaped sub-pubic angle
B. Deep and narrow greater sciatic notch
C. Large sacroiliac joint surface
D. Oval obturator foramen
E. Inverted ischial tuberosity
F. Prominent pre-auricular sulcus
a. ABCD b. ACDE
c. BCDE d. CDEF

Ans. c. BCDE

80. **Match the following with regard to fingerprints:**

A Permanent loss of fingerprints	1. Radiation burn
B. Retained pattern but change in gap between the ridges	2. Acromegaly
C. Complete loss of pattern with atrophy of ridges	3. Scleroderma
D. Incomplete ridge atrophy	4. Celiac disease
E. Ridge alteration	5. Dermatitis

a. A1, B2, C3, D4, E5
b. A2, B3, C5, D3, E1
c. A1, B2, C4, D5, E3
d. A4, B3, C1, D2, E5

Ans. c. A1, B2, C4, D5, E3

81. **A dye factory worker presented to ER with an alleged history of burning pain in the mouth, throat and abdomen, conjunctivitis, nausea and vomiting and dark loose stools. The suspected poisoning is:**

a. Lead
b. $KMnO_4$
c. Arsenic
d. Phosphorus

Ans. c. Arsenic

82. **The law/rules related to mental illness are:**

A. Ashley's law
B. Curren's rule
C. Murphy's law
D. Durham's rule

a. A and B
b. B and C
c. C and D
d. B and D

Ans. d. B and D

83. **Two friends consumed alcohol, after which they fought for a common girlfriend. One of them pushes the other onto the floor and covers his face/nose preventing him from breathing while sitting on his chest. This is known as:**

a. Traumatic asphyxia
b. Smothering
c. Burking
d. Overlaying

Ans. c. Burking

84. **A patient presented to OPD, with burns of soddened skin, with clear line of demarcation, lines of vesicles running down the body. The probable cause is:**

a. Chemical burn
b. Burn due to dry heat
c. Burn due to moist heat
d. Lightening

Ans. c. Burn due to moist heat

INI-CET JULY 2021

85. **Barberio's test detects:**

a. Choline
b. Spermine
c. Lecithin
d. Blood

Ans. b. Spermine

86. **Most common route of absorption of lead in case of industrial inorganic lead poisoning is by:**

a. Inhalation
b. Ingestion from contaminated hands
c. Skin contamination
d. Food contamination

Ans. a. Inhalation

87. **Identify the given image:**

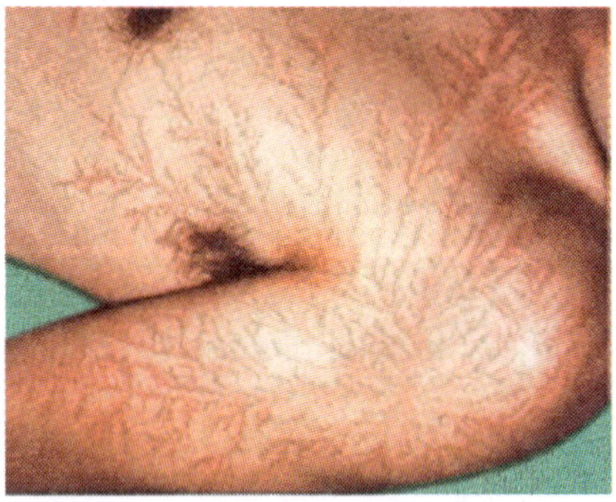

a. Postmortem lividity
b. Marbling
c. Filigree burns
d. None of the above

Ans c. Filigree burns

88. **A person arrested for murder was tortured by police by tying his hands and feet together behind his back. This is known as:**

a. Picana
b. Hog-tying
c. Ghotna
d. Falanga

Ans. b. Hog-tying

89. Match the following:

A. Fusion of lambdoid suture	i. 25 years
B. Fusion of basi-occiput	ii. 18-21 years
C. Fusion of medial end of clavicle	iii. 50-60 years
D. Body of sternum becomes a single bone	iv. 20-25 years

a. A-iii, B-ii, C-iv, D-i
b. A-i, B-iv, C-iii, D-ii
c. A-i, B-iii, C-iv, D-ii
d. A-iii, B-iv, C-ii, D-i

Ans. a. A-iii, B-ii, C-iv, D-i

90. Which of the following are features of female skull?

A. Prominent glabella
B. Prominent frontal eminence
C. Prominent parietal eminence
D. Round orbit
E. Prominent zygoma

a. A, B, C only
b. B, C, D only
c. B, D, E only
d. D only

Ans. b. B, C, D only

91. Which of the following are features of saltwater drowning?

A. Hyponatremia
B. Hypernatremia
C. Hemoconcentration
D. Hyperkalemia
E. Cardiac arrhythmia

a. A, B, C only
b. B, C, D only
c. B, D, E only
d. B, C only

Ans. d. B, C only

FMGE JULY 2023

92. A 10-year-old boy will have ____ permanent and ____ temporary teeth.

a. 20, 4
b. 16, 8
c. 12, 8
d. 12, 12

Ans. a. 20, 4

93. Identify the plant.

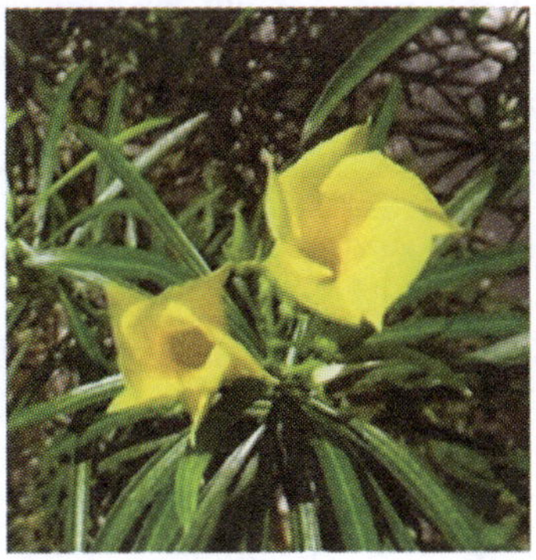

a. Nerium odorum
b. Cascabela thevetia
c. Aconite
d. Cerbera odollam

Ans. b. Cascabela thevetia

94. A dead body is brought for postmortem examination with stellate-shaped gunshot wound and muzzle impression print. What can be the distance?

a. Close range
b. Contact shot
c. Intermediate range
d. Distant range

Ans. b. Contact shot

95. A dead body is recovered from a river. The body has signs of antemortem drowning, and also has multiple cuts on flexor aspect of arm. What can be the cause of these wounds?

a. Self-inflicted wound
b. Active self-defense wound
c. Postmortem artifact
d. Passive self-defense wound

Ans. b. Active self-defense wound

96. MTP can be done up to 24 weeks for:

a. Contraceptive failure
b. Rape victim
c. Congenital malformation
d. Social indications

Ans. b. Rape victim

97. Patient died and relatives said he had a tattoo, but it was not visible on autopsy. Which is the best location of check for the evidence of tattoo?
    a. Spleen b. Artery
    c. Lymph node d. Liver

Ans. c. Lymph node

98. Police recovers beheaded skull. The relatives of a missing person give the photographs of missing person to police. These two samples can be analyzed with which technique?
    a. Fingerprint b. DNA fingerprint
    c. Superimposition d. Cheiloscopy

Ans. c. Superimposition

99. Case of road traffic accident presented with EDH. Where will be impact of collision?
    a. Pterion
    b. Angle of mandible
    c. Lambdoid suture
    d. None of the above

Ans. a. Pterion

FMGE JANUARY 2023

100. Study of death in all its aspects is called:
    a. Thanatopraxia b. Disinterment
    c. Thanatology d. Molecular death

Ans. c. Thanatology

101. Cherry red postmortem hypostasis is seen in:
    a. Carbon monoxide
    b. Hydrogen sulfide
    c. Yellow phosphorus
    d. Hydrogen cyanide

Ans. a. Carbon monoxide

102. On examination of a dead body, there was stiffness of one group of muscles absence of primary relaxation. What is true about this?
    a. Algor mortis b. Livor mortis
    c. Rigor mortis d. Cadaveric spasm

Ans. d. Cadaveric spasm

103. In case of death in police custody, the inquest is held by:
    a. Jail Superintendent
    b. Executive Magistrate
    c. Police Inspector
    d. Judicial Magistrate

Ans. d. Judicial Magistrate

104. Police recovers a skull in the forest and the relatives of a missing person give his photograph to police. These two can be analyzed with which technique:
    a. Fingerprint
    b. DNA fingerprint
    c. Superimposition
    d. Cheiloscopy

Ans. c. Superimposition

105. Combination of homicidal smothering and traumatic asphyxia is cause of death in:
    a. Burking b. Bansdola
    c. Mugging d. Garroting

Ans. a. Burking

106. "To establish a defense on the ground of insanity, it must be clearly shown that at the time of committing the act, the accused was laboring under such a defect of reason, from disease of mind, as not to know the nature and quality of the act he was doing or, if he did know it, that he did not know that what he was doing was wrong." This is according to which Law of insanity:
    a. M'Naghten rule
    b. Durham law
    c. Curren's rule
    d. Irresistible impulse test

Ans. a. M'Naghten rule

107. Which of the following is not a blood stain analysis test?
    a. Barberio's
    b. Teichmann's
    c. Takayama hemochromogen
    d. Spectroscopy

Ans. a. Barberio's

108. A 10-year-old child has consumed lots of iron tablets in home and brought in casualty with features of abdominal pain, profound gastrointestinal bleeding episodes and is lethargic. Preferred treatment in this case is:
   a. Deferoxamine mesylate
   b. Penicillamine
   c. BAL
   d. Activated charcoal

Ans. a. Deferoxamine mesylate

109. All of the following are the signs and symptoms of acute cocaine poisoning during the stage of excitement; EXCEPT:
   a. Feeling of well-being
   b. Tingling or numbness in hands and feet
   c. Pupils dilated and rapid pulse and sweating
   d. Cocaine bugs

Ans. d. Cocaine bugs

FMGE MAY 2022

110. Sexual pleasure obtained by getting hurt by opposite sex is called:
   a. Masochism
   b. Sadism
   c. Transvestism
   d. Exhibitionism

Ans. a. Masochism

111. As per MTP Act 2021, opinion of 2 doctors is required for:
   a. 12–20 weeks pregnancy
   b. 20–24 weeks pregnancy
   c. 12–24 weeks pregnancy
   d. 20–26 weeks pregnancy

Ans. b. 20–24 weeks pregnancy

112. Artificial bruise can be differentiated from true bruise by which of the following?
   a. Presence of vesicles
   b. Color change noted with time
   c. Diffuse irregular margins
   d. No itching

Ans. a. Presence of vesicles

113. Grievous hurt is said to be there if the person is in severe body pain/unable to follow ordinary pursuits for minimum of how many days:
   a. 6 b. 18
   c. 20 d. 25

Ans. c. 20

114. Which test is used to differentiate species of a blood sample whether sample belongs to human or animal?
   a. Teichmann's test
   b. Takayama's test
   c. DNA-based method
   d. Barberio's test

Ans. c. DNA-based method

115. A substance abuser was found on roadside with pinpoint pupils. Which of the following should be suspected?
   a. Morphine b. Cocaine
   c. Alcohol d. Cyanide

Ans. a. Morphine

116. In an injury, it is noted under microscope that hair bulbs were crushed. Most likely the injury is:
   a. Abrasion
   b. Incised wound
   c. Lacerated wound
   d. Stab wound

Ans. c. Lacerated wound

117. In court of law, examination of a witness is being done to develop new and old facts and try to weaken the evidence by showing that evidence was biased, inaccurate, inconsistent by lawyer during which of the following?
   a. Direct examination
   b. Cross examination
   c. Redirect examination
   d. Court room examination

Ans. b. Cross examination

118. A patient died because of doctor's negligence but some other factors of the patient were also present for the reason of death. This kind of malpractice is known as:
   a. Contributory negligence
   b. Res ipsa loquitor
   c. Volenti non fit injuria
   d. Respondeat superior

Ans. a. Contributory negligence

119. A person was brought to OPD with history of snake bite 8 hours ago. Patient was noted to be in respiratory depression with HR-50/min. along with drooping of eyelids bilaterally. 10 vials of polyvalent antivenom was administered. No ventilator was available in the hospital. What is the next management?
   a. Give atropine + neostigmine
   b. Check for blood coagulation profile
   c. IV Hydrocortisone
   d. Inj. Epinephrine

Ans. a. Give atropine + neostigmine

120. A child with leg weakness is brought to the OPD. The blood lead level is 60 mcg/100 mL. The treatment is:
   a. BAL + EDTA
   b. Deferoxamine
   c. Prussian blue
   d. Penicillamine

Ans. a. BAL + EDTA

121. Among the following which has highest affinity for hemoglobin?
   a. Carbon monoxide
   b. Oxygen
   c. Nitrogen
   d. Carbon di oxide

Ans. a. Carbon monoxide

FMGE DECEMBER 2021

122. What type of toxin is released by the snake shown below?

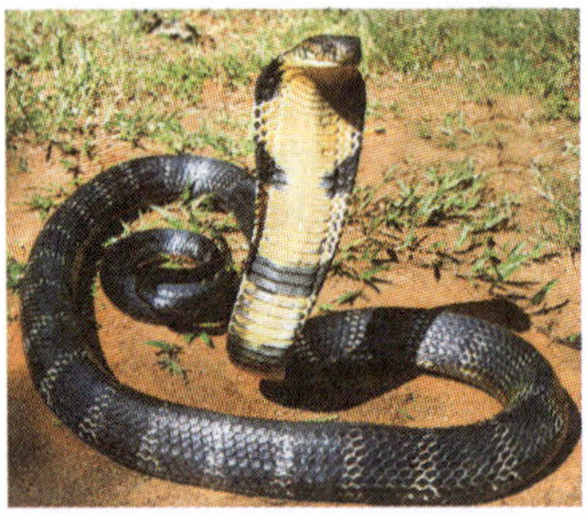

   a. Hematotoxin
   b. Myotoxin
   c. Neurotoxin
   d. Vasculotoxic

Ans. c. Neurotoxin

123. A patient was referred by a doctor to a radiologist for CT scan. Radiologist gave commission to the doctor. It is described as:
   a. Dichotomy
   b. Covering
   c. Canvassing
   d. Association

Ans. a. Dichotomy

124. A man was brought to the hospital with uncontrolled excessive sexual desire. Which of the following could the man be suffering from?
   a. Satyriasis
   b. Nymphomania
   c. Necromania
   d. Fetichism

Ans. a. Satyriasis

125. Identify the plant shown in the image below:

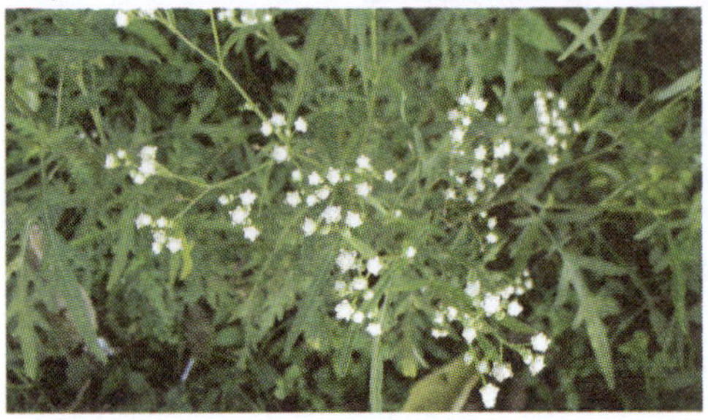

   a. Calotropis
   b. Parthenium
   c. Cannabis
   d. Chrysanthemum

Ans. b. Parthenium

126. Which of the following is the true statement for the given image?

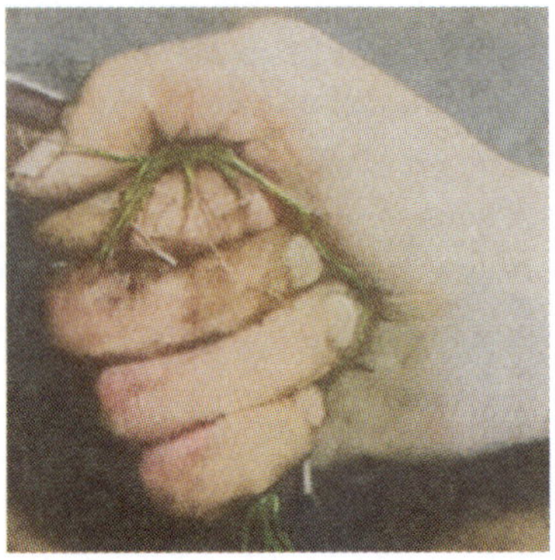

   a. A case of homicide
   b. A case of suicide
   c. Rigor mortis
   d. Cadaveric spasm

Ans. d. Cadaveric spasm

127. An image is given below. Identify the odor caused by it:

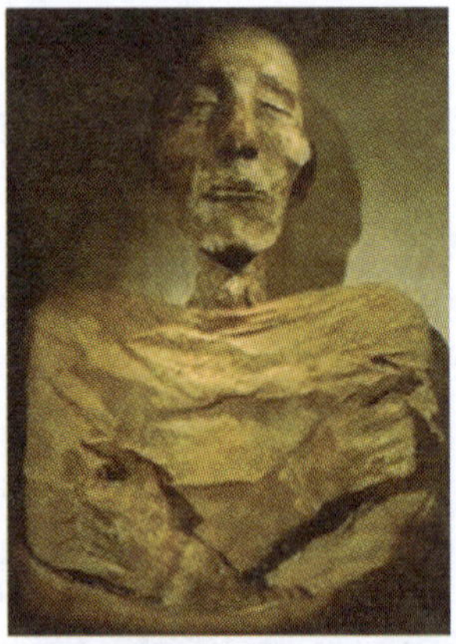

a. Ammoniacal
b. Odorless
c. Foul
d. Rancid

Ans. b. Odorless

128. Identify the postmortem finding:

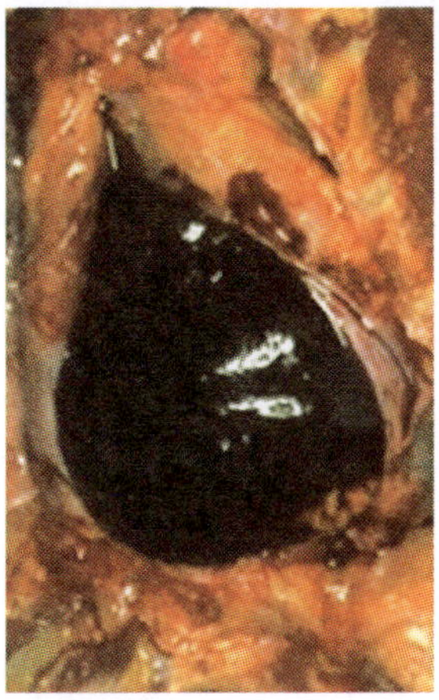

a. Left lung missing
b. Fat necrosis
c. Cardiac tamponade
d. Pulmonary embolism

Ans. c. Cardiac tamponade

129. Identify the blood test shown in the image below:

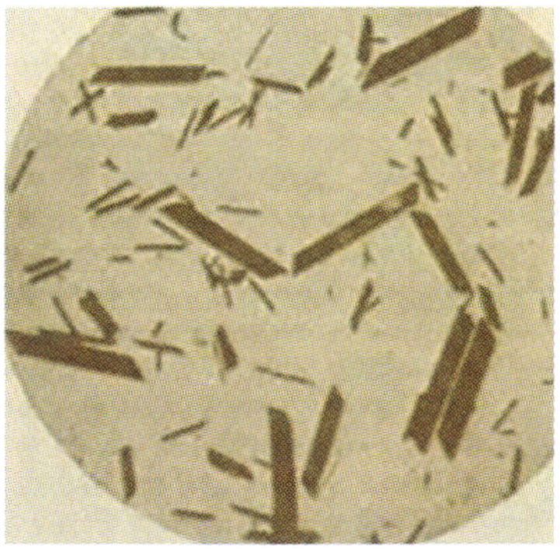

a. Barberio's test
b. Florence test
c. Takayama's test
d. Teichmann's test

Ans. d. Teichmann's test

130. A patient who took an unknown poison brought to the hospital. On examination, there was excessive sweating, lacrimation, bradycardia. Blood pressure was 80/60 mm Hg. Which of the following antidote should be given?

a. Diazepam
b. Atropine
c. Oximes
d. Naloxone

Ans. b. Atropine

131. Lucid interval is most commonly seen in:

a. Subdural hemorrhage
b. Extradural hemorrhage
c. Subarachnoid hemorrhage
d. Intracranial hemorrhage

Ans. b. Extradural hemorrhage

132. Battle sign is seen in:

a. Fracture of anterior cranial fossa
b. Fracture of middle cranial fossa
c. Ring fracture
d. Fracture of posterior cranial fossa

Ans. b. Fracture of middle cranial fossa

133. A couple did not want a girl child and aborted by using an abnormal method. What could be the method used for criminal abortion?

a. Vacuum aspiration
b. Prostaglandins
c. Dilatation and curettage
d. Abortion stick

Ans. d. Abortion stick

FMGE JULY 2021

134. Gutter fracture of skull is associated with:

a. Sharp object
b. Blunt object
c. Fall from height
d. Bullet

Ans. d. Bullet

135. Cherry red colored PM lividity is associated with poisoning by:

a. Hydrogen sulfide
b. Hydrocyanic acid
c. Carbon monoxide
d. Nitrites

Ans. c. Carbon monoxide

136. In Barberio's test, yellow needle-shaped crystals are seen under microscope. This is done to detect:

a. Saliva
b. Semen
c. Blood
d. CSF

Ans. b. Semen

137. A 42-year-old patient was brought to the casualty. At the time of the presentation, he was unconscious. He was presented because of unknown poisoning. On examination, it was seen that there were some needle track ulcers on the upper limb. He had increased blood pressure and heart rate. Which of the following poisoning can be expected?
   a. Heroin b. Cocaine
   c. LSD d. Cannabis

Ans. b. Cocaine

138. A person met with an accident and he was taken by the local people to the hospital. He was not accompanied by any of his relatives or friends. As the condition of the patient was bad, the doctors have to suggest him emergency surgery. According to ethics, What should be done?
   a. Doctor can do the surgery in the case of emergency
   b. Has to wait for getting consent from his relatives
   c. Has to wait for the consent of the hospital administrators
   d. Has to get consent from the police station

Ans. a. Doctor can do the surgery in the case of emergency

139. A farmer was brought to the casualty with pinpoint pupil, increased secretions and garlicky odor from the breath. The ideal antidote for poisoning is:
   a. Oximes b. Atropine
   c. Physostigmine d. N-acetyl cysteine

Ans. b. Atropine

140. Judicial hanging is the method of execution of a condemned criminal in our country. The cause of death in such cases would be:
   a. Vagal inhibition
   b. Fracture dislocation of cervical vertebrae
   c. Cerebral hypoxia
   d. Asphyxia

Ans. b. Fracture dislocation of cervical vertebrae

141. A 35-year-old person comes to the casualty with a history of consumption of some unknown seeds. On examination, there was dilated pupil, dry mouth and decreased secretions. The suspected poisoning is by:
   a. Cocaine b. Cannabis
   c. Heroin d. Datura

Ans. d. Datura

142. First tooth to appear is:
   a. Lower central incisor
   b. Upper central incisor
   c. First molar
   d. None of the above

Ans. a. Lower central incisor

143. A person who has committed a crime has been brought before the court of law by the police. The court may direct the police to take him to the Juvenile court, if his age is:
   a. 17 years b. 19 years
   c. 20 years d. None of these

Ans. a. 17 years

144. A person died due to chronic starvation. The true finding is:
   a. Expanded lungs
   b. Enlarged heart
   c. Enlarged stomach
   d. Distended gallbladder

Ans. d. Distended gallbladder

145. A child consumes iron tablets used by its mother. The antidote is:
   a. BAL b. EDTA
   c. Deferoxamine d. Trientine

Ans. c. Deferoxamine

146. Partial hanging may resemble strangulation by:
   a. Knot mark
   b. Situation below the thyroid cartilage
   c. Dribbling of saliva
   d. Transverse ligature mark

Ans. d. Transverse ligature mark